Living Wills and More

Everything You Need to Ensure That All Your Medical Wishes Are Followed

TERRY J. BARNETT

JOHN WILEY & SONS, INC.

New York / Chichester / Brisbane / Toronto / Singapore

In memory of my parents,
Saul and Idelle Barnett.

In recognition of the importance of preserving what has been written, it is a policy of John Wiley & Sons, Inc., to have books of enduring value printed on acid-free paper, and we exert our best efforts to that end.

This publication is designed to provide accurate and authoritative information in regard to the subject matter covered. It is sold with the understanding that the publisher is not engaged in rendering legal, accounting, or other professional service. If legal advice or other expert assistance is required, the services of a competent professional person should be sought. From a *Declaration of Principles jointly adopted by a Committee of the American Bar Association and a Committee of Publishers.*

Library of Congress Cataloging-in-Publication Data

Barnett, Terry J.
  Living wills and more / Terry J. Barnett.
      p.   cm.
      Includes index.
      ISBN 0-471-57394-9 (paper)
      1. Right to die—Law and legislation—United States—Popular
  works.   2. Power of attorney—United States—Popular works.
  I. Title.
  KF3827.E87B37   1993
  344.73′04197—dc20
  [347.3044197]   92-19626

CONTENTS

The timing of death—once a matter of fate—is now a matter of human choice.
— Office of Technology Assessment Task Force, *Life Sustaining Technology and the Elderly* (1988), quoted by the United States Supreme Court in *Cruzan v. Director, Missouri Department of Health* (1990)

There are some things we might rather not be a matter of choice, but modern medicine has laid the choice of the timing of death before us, by developing treatments that can sustain life that some judge not worth living. The ability to sustain life is not bad; what one person sees as living death another might see as a gift of life. The problem is to use such power in a way that respects the person whom treatment is supposed to benefit.

The ability to suspend death challenges us morally, as a society and as individuals. One way our society is responding is by legally empowering people to reject life-sustaining treatment they do not want. Starting in 1976, states began to pass laws that authorize living wills, documents that instruct physicians to stop, or not to start, life-sustaining treatment in certain circumstances. Then in 1983, states began to provide for durable powers of attorney for health-care decisions, documents that name representatives to make health-care decisions for those who later become unable to do so personally. Powers of attorney can also give guidance for decision making.

As with medical treatment tools, we have a lot to learn about how to use these health-care planning documents. A persistent mistake, made not only by laypeople but also by health-care providers, has been to treat health-care planning rights, laws, and documents as substitutes for communication. Consequently, documents often haven't worked very well, for anyone concerned.

This book has two messages. First, health-care planning documents need to do much more than just meet legal requirements; they need to explain your intentions and choices in ways that your health-care providers, family, and representative can understand and accept. Second, while having good documents is important, what you *do* with your documents can be even more important. Decisions about use of life-sustaining treatment almost always involve deeply felt, and sometimes conflicting, values and feelings. A document alone might not address them to the satisfaction of everyone who cares about you. For the sake of all concerned, you need to discuss your intentions face to face. A good document can guide you through that discussion.

This book provides ready-to-use model documents along with step-by-step instructions and advice on how to use them to maximize the likelihood that they will work as and when you intend. It also provides important information about common life-sustaining medical treatments, to help you decide what choices are right for you and to aid discussion about your intentions with health-care providers and other people who are concerned about your care.

The model documents have been carefully designed to be as comprehensive, clear, and persuasive as possible, for laypeople, health-care providers, lawyers, and courts. They reflect three years of experience with people in different states of health, work with hospital ethics committees on cases and policies involving life-sustaining treatment, and lots of listening to the concerns of health-care providers and consumers. They have been tested with nearly 1,000 people during that time to help make them as useful as possible for health-care planning, particularly avoiding unwanted life-sustaining treatment.

Chapter 1 provides basic information about living wills and health-care durable powers of attorney. Chapter 2 explains why health-care providers, families, and representatives can have trouble understanding and accepting intentions to stop, or not to start, life-sustaining treatment, and advises how to talk with them about their concerns. Chapter 3 answers questions you might have about health-care planning documents. Chapter 4 introduces a model health-care durable power of attorney and model living will. Chapter 5 explains the model documents section by section, and provides basic medical information to help you talk with your health-care providers about your intentions and make decisions about use of life-sustaining treatment. Chapter 6 addresses legal requirements you need to be aware of for the state where you live. The model documents and any related state documents you might need appear in the appendixes.

If the quality of your life is more important to you than its duration, and you want decisions about your health care to be based on your choices even if you become unable to speak for yourself, then this book is for you.

REQUEST FOR READER RESPONSE

Health-care advocates, planners, policy makers, providers, researchers, and others are devoting a lot of effort to health-care planning issues. Particular concerns for me are what providers and laypeople want health-care planning documents to say, and whether and how documents affect the process of decision making about use of life-sustaining treatment, from the perspectives of everyone involved.

Whether your involvement has been as a prospective or actual patient, a family member, an agent, a health-care provider, a friend, or more than one of those, I would welcome hearing about your experiences, both good and bad. How did the model documents, or other documents, suit you (whether they were yours or someone else's)? Were the models changed in some way to reflect the maker's personal preferences or needs, or issues raised by a physician or someone else? If so, what changes were made? How did the discussion suggestions in this book work for you? Were intentions and choices expressed in documents respected, and why? Whatever your part in the process, did you feel able to contribute, listened to, and respected?

Correspondence can be sent to:

Terry J. Barnett,
c/o Royalty Department
John Wiley & Sons, Inc.
605 Third Avenue
New York, NY 10158-0012

ACKNOWLEDGMENTS

Many people have contributed to this book. Clients with whom I worked to make health-care planning documents shared their feelings with me, and their questions helped me shape what became the model documents this book offers. My colleagues on the ethics committees at the Group Health Cooperative of Puget Sound (Seattle, Washington), the Veterans Administration Medical Center (Seattle, Washington) and Western State Hospital (Fort Steilacoom, Washington) all influenced my understanding of vital issues, from several perspectives. Jonathan D. Mayer, Ph.D., of the University of Washington, encouraged my early interest in medical ethics and became an important colleague. Albert R. Jonsen, Ph.D., chair of the Department of Medical History and Ethics at the University of Washington, welcomed me into activities of the department. Thomas R. McCormick, D.Sc., senior lecturer in medical ethics at the University of Washington, contributed vitally to my understanding of how physicians and nurses see and handle dilemmas in use of life-sustaining treatment. Fellow Group Health Ethics Committee members Janice C. Benson, M.D. and John F. Howe, M.D.; Dr. Mayer, Michael W. Baker, Ph.D.; and my wife, Rebecca M. G. Barnett each made important contributions to the book draft. I owe very special thanks and enormous gratitude to Dr. Baker, executive director of the Dorothy Garske Center (Phoenix, Arizona); the opportunity to develop health-care planning documents and legislation for the center, and to work with him over a period of nearly two years, contributed immensely to this book. David A. Smith, director of legal services, and William Prip, legal assistant, at Choice in Dying in New York City very helpfully provided the latest information about which states had enacted new laws or amended existing ones. I want to thank Senior Editor Steve Ross for his faith in this project, and both him and Assistant Editor Judith McCarthy for their significant editorial contributions. Finally, and most of all, I want to thank my wife so much for her encouragement and support.

CHAPTER 1

Basic Information on Living Wills and Durable Powers of Attorney for Health Care

Modern medicine can seem miraculous. Conditions that even recently were untreatable have become preventable, manageable, and even curable. Remarkable progress undoubtedly will continue. Still, throughout history, medicine has had limits. Now the most troublesome limits are technical and moral.

Technical limits concern whether a medical goal *can* be accomplished. For example, can an antibiotic cure a pneumonia? Can heart function be restored after a heart attack occurs? Moral limits concern whether a technically achievable medical goal *should* be pursued. Should a pneumonia be treated, or should cardiopulmonary resuscitation be attempted, if a person is so debilitated that technical success will leave her bedridden, ventilator-dependent, and unable to communicate, for probably only a few more days or weeks of life? Who should answer such questions, and how?

Because of the power of medical techniques, such questions are decided every day for literally thousands of people. These are not medical questions, to which there are objective answers; they are moral issues.

Morality is not a matter of expertise; neither training nor experience equips physicians and nurses to make moral decisions for their patients. Health-care providers can give important technical information to help in making such decisions. They also might be able to give personal advice, especially if they know a patient well. But they cannot know whether the life that medicine can sustain is worth living.

Until fairly recently in medical history, the technical and moral aims of medicine met in a common goal: to preserve life. The moral validity of preserving life was unquestioned, in part because medicine lacked the ability to sustain a life that anyone would consider not worth living. The only decisions to be made were technical, so physicians were the natural decision makers.

The revolution in medical technique has broken the seamless connection between physicians' and patients' goals. Now life can be sustained—sometimes for years—in conditions that many people consider worse than death. Because of that threat, many people are becoming more concerned about their quality of life than simply its duration.

Except in rare circumstances, the ultimate decision maker should be the person whose life is in question, or someone that person has entrusted to decide for him if he becomes unable to speak personally. But many people—laypeople and health-care providers alike—do not really accept the idea that decisions about the use of medical tools should depend on patients' values. Even people who do can still feel intense pressure to extend life as long as possible. One of the most powerful stresses can be uncertainty about just what a person would truly want when a decision is being made for him. Two major reasons for that uncertainty are weakened relationships between physicians and patients, and weakened relationships within families.

As medical technology has changed so have physician-patient relationships. Not so long ago patients and physicians often built trusting relationships over many years; now, many people don't have a regular physician. When physicians and patients do meet, the experience is not what it once was. Diagnosis and treatment used to mean a physician spending time with a patient, listening, talking, and touching. Now a large part of diagnosis consists of testing, often conducted by a specialist physician or by a technician whom the patient doesn't know. Treatments, too, often are administered by strangers—or, as more conditions become treatable by medications, by patients themselves. Too often, physicians and patients don't talk as much as they should.

Family relationships are changing, too. Family members often live far apart, making it difficult for them to be present to give emotional support and make decisions during an illness, especially one that continues for long. They may be less likely than in the past to hold the same personal values about what makes life worth living. When family members are unsure about each other's values, or when they know their values differ, they may feel unable to make major medical decisions, especially decisions that result in death. The knowledge that families do not necessarily share basic values can make physicians hesitant to accept their decisions to limit life-sustaining treatment. Doubts can weigh even more heavily when a physician feels the patient would want such treatment, or when he personally feels such treatment should be used.

All of these influences—depersonalization of physician-patient relationships, geographic and value dispersal of families, and especially expansion of life-support capability—have eroded traditional faith in medical decision making. As a society we have tried to shore up weakened trust with the legal timbers of patient rights and provider duties. Primary among these is the right of every competent adult (and sometimes minors) to consent, refuse consent, or withdraw consent already given, for medical procedures that health-care providers offer, and the duty of providers to respect those choices. An important expression of that right is health-care planning documents.

Unfortunately, the legal principle of self-determination and its expression in health-care planning documents often conflict with ingrained medical values. Physicians see themselves as responsible for protecting patients from "bad" decisions. Decisions may be seen as "bad" when they are based on information that is incomplete, or on "emotional" considerations. In the views of many physicians, the factual basis of a health-care planning document made when a person is healthy necessarily is unacceptably incomplete. Also, physicians may see laypeople's quality of life choices as emotional rather than rational. Many providers see health-care values and patient rights laws as fundamentally incompatible. The problem does not rest just with providers; patient rights laws often are insensitive to their legitimate concerns. This is one reason it so important that you plan ahead to build support for your intentions.

SECURING YOUR HEALTH-CARE CHOICES

Think about what you would and would not want from health care if you were to experience a life-threatening condition. You would want to be treated with respect, to be cured if possible, but always to be cared for. You would want peace of mind, for yourself and for those who care about you. You would not want your providers, your family, or your representative to feel compelled to continue life-sustaining treatment because when they find themselves facing a decision they realize they don't know what you would want. You would not want your family or physicians or nurses to oppose your wishes because of personal values, misunderstanding, or emotional confusion that makes them feel they must do everything possible. And, you would not want anyone to end up in court. That is why it is so important for you to document your intentions in a way that is sensitive to your providers' and family members' concerns, and to use your documents to build understanding and acceptance of your choices.

Documents work when they accomplish your intentions with the least stress for all concerned. How can you reach that goal?

Protecting your health-care choices is a three-step process: *deciding* what you want, *communicating* your intentions so that others understand them, and *committing* your providers, family, and representative to the acceptance (and sometimes defense) of your choices.

Deciding What You Want

You need to be clear in your own mind about your intentions. That might seem obvious, but many people think they are clear when they are not. Some people say, for example, that they don't ever want life-sustaining treatment, when they really *do* want such treatment if it will help them recover from illness or injury; what they want to avoid is being sustained indefinitely in a debilitated condition. The medical information and the discussion process presented in this book can help you clarify your intentions.

Communicating Your Intentions

This book shows you how to communicate your intentions by documenting them, and then using your documents to guide discussion with your family, providers, and representative.

Your documents need to be specific about what you want and when. The terms you use to express your intentions should mean the same thing to others as they do to you. Words such as "hopeless," "extraordinary," "ordinary," "meaningful," "extreme," "reasonable," "invasive," and "heroic" should be avoided because they are vague. So too are "relatively short time" and "reasonably short period of time"—phrases that appear in many living will laws.

Similarly, terms such as "terminal," "incurable," and "irreversible," which have clearer meanings but cover a wide range of time and circumstances, can leave providers and family paralyzed with doubts about when, and what, treatments to use or not use. Some conditions that are terminal, incurable, and irreversible can develop for years before quality of life is severely impaired or death results. Faced with an immediate threat to life from some other cause, one person with such a disorder might not want any life-sustaining treatment even if the condition has not yet progressed to the point of serious disability. Another person might want everything done until disability reaches a certain stage. Someone else might want certain life-sustaining treatments but not others. Some people might want everything to be done for as long as possible. If your providers and family aren't sure what you intend, they will have to guess what you would want, or decide what to do based on what is important to them. That can be hard on them, and on you.

The model documents in Appendixes A and B are designed to help you communicate your wishes effectively. Pertinent information, issues, and approaches are discussed throughout the book.

Building Commitment

The model documents are designed in part to serve as a map for discussion with your family, your providers, and your representatives (your primary one, and an alternate), to try to build understanding and acceptance of your choices. Why are discussions necessary? Documents that seem clear, and are legal, often fail to work because family or health-care providers are not willing to accept them.

Why would family and providers resist your choices? The very simple answer is: they don't want to lose you. No matter how clearly and personally a document speaks, they may need to hear from *you*. And they, in turn, need you to hear and acknowledge *their* concerns.

Many people assume that because health-care planning documents are legal providers and family have to follow them, so there's no need for discussion. The reality, though, is that such documents operate first, and usually only, in health-care settings, where legal values usually are considered less important than medical ones. Also, in most states the law expressly excuses physicians and nurses from accepting patient choices to which they object for reasons of conscience. Similarly, in some states the law excuses health-care facilities from honoring choices that conflict with institutional policy. In a few cases, courts have forced facilities to accept patient choices. Individual physicians may also be required to do so, when transfer to another provider who will accept the patient's choice is not feasible. But when treatment disputes end up in court everyone loses, especially patients and families. Legal actions can be terribly costly, both emotionally and financially. And, while a case is in court (which can stretch to a year or more), unwanted treatment continues. Good documents, thoughtfully used to build a foundation for acceptance, can help you, your family, and your providers avoid a lot of pain.

YOUR OPTIONS

There are two widely accepted kinds of documents for guiding health-care decisions if you become unable to make them personally: the durable power of attorney for health care, and the directive or declaration to physicians (often called a "living will").

A directive or declaration is a document in which you instruct physicians not to start life-sustaining treatment, or to stop such treatment already in use, in circumstances the document describes.

The durable power of attorney is a document by which you can transfer certain legal authority to someone else to exercise for you. "Durable" means the document can operate if you become physically or mentally unable to make decisions personally. So, a durable power of attorney for health care is a document that empowers a person you choose to make health-care decisions (not limited to use of life-sustaining treatment) for you if you become unable to do so for yourself. The laws in New York and Massachusetts call a health-care power of attorney a "health-care proxy." The New Jersey law uses the term "proxy directive" as well as "durable power of attorney."

The person a health-care power of attorney names to make decisions is usually called an "agent," so this book will use that term. Some laws call an agent an "attorney in fact," but an agent does not have to be an attorney. Sometimes an agent is called a "proxy." The law in Michigan calls an agent a "patient advocate," in Florida a "surrogate," and in West Virginia a "representative." In Arizona both "agent" and "surrogate" are used.

Your state may have a law that authorizes certain people to make health-care decisions for you if you become incapacitated even if you have not made a health-care planning document. The law calls these people "surrogates" or "proxies." While authorizing decision makers, such laws don't help them know what *you* would want. So, even in states that have surrogate laws it is a good idea to make health-care planning documents.

Currently, most state laws that authorize surrogate decision makers do not require that surrogates act according to the patient's known wishes, even if these wishes are expressed in a living will. Such laws, however, usually give an agent named in a health-care durable power of attorney priority over all other potential surrogates (except a guardian appointed by court order). So, in these states as elsewhere, you can help protect your choices by making a health-care durable power of attorney if an appropriate agent is available (see Chapter 3, Question 15, pp. 25–27).

In most states the laws that authorize directives or declarations include a document form, and in a few of these states the form has a space for naming a health-care agent. There is nothing wrong with naming an agent in a living will, but living wills are weak means for expressing health-care choices. For that reason, if you have access to an appropriate agent you should make a health-care power of attorney even if you also name an agent in a living will.

The Legal Status of Living Wills and Health-Care Durable Powers of Attorney

Living wills and health-care durable powers of attorney have legal status in every state, although that status is not the same everywhere.

Declarations and directives are authorized by law in the District of Columbia and every state except Massachusetts, Michigan, and New York (as of December 31, 1992). They may have legal power even in these states. Important features of the law in each state and the District of Columbia are addressed in Chapter 6.

Durable powers of attorney for health care have legal standing in nearly every state. Many states have special health-care power of attorney laws. Other states have general power of attorney laws (mainly concerned with authority over property) that are usually broad enough to include health-care decision making.

Besides legal status, official statements of major physician organizations support the use of health-care planning documents, and doctors may honor them for that reason.

Important Differences between the Types of Documents

There are important differences between directives or declarations to physicians and health-care durable powers of attorney, in terms of both how they work and how well they can be expected to work.

A directive or declaration speaks directly to providers, and the laws that authorize them contain restrictions about when they can be honored and the kinds of choices providers can accept. A power of attorney authorizes an agent to speak for you with your providers, and usually allow your agent to make every kind of decision for you that you could make yourself if you were acting in person.

Directives and declarations to physicians are weak means for health-care planning because they can involve serious medical, legal, ethical, and personal value uncertainties, and there may be no one to

speak with sufficient authority for you to resolve such questions. If you have only a directive or declaration, a physician who wants to respect your choices can feel prevented by uncertainty or opposition from a family member or another provider; a physician who believes that doctors should make all treatment decisions can evade your intentions. Realistically, obstacles to acceptance of living wills are so significant that such documents are better thought of as "living wishes." A health-care durable power of attorney has the advantage of giving discretionary authority to someone you know and trust to act in your place. It addresses uncertainty and opposition by giving your agent authority to make (and, if necessary, push) decisions for you whatever the circumstances.

Most physicians prefer powers of attorney to directives or declarations, in part because a power of attorney appoints a person with whom a physician can talk personally, just as she would with the patient, about actual, existing medical facts and options. The model durable power of attorney is designed in part to give your physician confidence in your agent's choices, by explaining your intentions and the reasons behind them.

The Problem of Restrictions on Choice

Nearly every law that authorizes directives or declarations limits withholding and withdrawing life-sustaining treatment to "terminal conditions." Further, many of these laws specify that death from a terminal condition must be imminent, or be expected to occur in a "relatively short time" or "reasonably short period of time." Many laws consider a condition not to be terminal whenever death can be delayed by life-sustaining treatment. Limitations of this kind can be misused to justify imposing life support on almost everyone who will eventually die from a chronic illness. In fact, permanent unconsciousness—a condition in which most people do not want to be sustained—legally is not a terminal condition in many states. (The exceptions are noted in Chapter 6, Table 2, and the list is growing.) Terminal condition limitations undermine the basic reason people make health-care planning documents: to avoid prolonging their dying.

Imminent death provisions also contradict the reason that most people make health-care planning documents. There are two types of "imminent death" provisions. One type says that death must be imminent if life support is not used—in other words, that death will occur shortly if life support is not started or is stopped. The other type says that death is not considered imminent as long as a person can be kept alive by life support. Under this type, a directive or declaration would almost never apply, because life-sustaining treatment would have to be started whenever it could sustain life, and be continued until a physician decided that death was imminent.

"Imminent" has no particular medical or legal meaning. Neither does "relatively short time" or "reasonably short period of time." "Terminal condition" is usually defined in living will laws, but the legal definitions are often not familiar, or useful, to physicians. In practice such terms can confuse physicians about when they can honor a directive or declaration. The vagueness of these limitations can also allow a physician who wants to avoid a directive or declaration to do so.

Many states also limit the kinds of life-sustaining treatment that can be stopped or not started based on a living will, particularly artificial nutrition and hydration (see pp. 50–51 for discussion of these terms). Recently, several states have abandoned restrictions on artificial nutrition and hydration in favor of treating those measures the same as other life-sustaining treatments. Whether other states will follow remains to be seen.

Many laws also exclude medications from treatments that can be rejected by living wills. Some do so clearly, while others are vague about whether all medications are excluded or only medications used for pain relief.

Finally, most living will laws suspend treatment refusal during pregnancy. Most pregnancy exclusions state either that treatment refusal documents do not apply at any time during pregnancy, or that they do not apply if use of life support could permit a fetus to develop to birth. State pregnancy exclusions are listed in Chapter 6, Table 3. Such restrictions probably violate the federal constitutional right to avoid unwanted life-sustaining treatment, and may violate other legal rights. If this issue concerns you, you should discuss it with your agents, physician, and family. If you are a woman of childbearing age and you are using a state form with a pregnancy restriction that you do not want, cross it out.

Some health-care power of attorney laws contain restrictions similar to those in living will laws. The laws in Nebraska and Ohio state that an agent cannot consent to withholding and withdrawing life-sustaining treatment unless the person whose life is in question has a terminal condition or is permanently unconscious. That may be so in

Tennessee as well (the law is not clear). In Utah there is a limitation to terminal condition without mention of permanent unconsciousness. In several other states (Alaska, California, the District of Columbia, Florida, Georgia, Nevada, New Hampshire, Oklahoma, Oregon, Texas, Vermont, Virginia, Washington, Wisconsin, and Wyoming) the laws prohibit agents from consenting to psychiatric confinement and treatment, surgery, abortion, and/or sterilization; these procedures require a court order. A few power of attorney laws have pregnancy restrictions (see Chapter 6, Table 3).

Legally, you are probably entitled to avoid any medical treatment you do not want, no matter what your condition, despite limitations in these laws. Many of the laws, themselves, state that they intend only to provide one means to avoid unwanted treatment, not to restrict other such rights. These include the right of personal liberty in the United States Constitution, and the right of bodily integrity under the common law. (Common law is a body of basic rights and obligations developed over time by courts.) But exactly how these various rights fit together remains to be seen. Legal uncertainty is one reason it is so important to have the support of your physician and your family.

Overcoming Restrictive Laws

Legal uncertainty can make physicians afraid to withhold or stop life-sustaining treatment. Physicians may think that the law requires or prohibits something, but not be sure and not get legal advice. When they do seek advice, what they hear can make the situation worse. Lawyers whom physicians consult about patient care issues usually work for hospitals or other health-care facilities. They tend to take a restrictive view of patient rights when they think that best serves institutional interests, and they advise physicians accordingly. In the real world of medical decision making, legal fears can make providers feel unable to act on patients' intentions. Sometimes, though, physicians overlook restrictive laws and legal advice, out of respect and compassion for their patients. Whether that happens depends largely on the quality of communication that takes place among patients, physicians, family members, and agents in the health-care planning process.

In summary, living wills and durable powers of attorney differ in these ways:

- A health-care durable power of attorney
  (1) appoints an agent you choose to make health-care decisions for you if you become unable to make decisions personally
  (2) usually permits an agent to make all health-care decisions in all circumstances, unless your document expressly provides otherwise
  (3) should direct your agent to make decisions as you would make them yourself, or, if what you would want is not known, then as the agent believes is in your best interest (based on personal knowledge of you and on information and advice from your physician)
- A living will
  (1) effectively leaves decision making up to your physicians (especially if you have no family, or if they cannot act strongly for you)
  (2) is basically limited to refusal of unwanted life-sustaining treatment, and

may be interpreted as being subject to other restrictions

(3) can be inflexible and confusing about the circumstances in which it applies, and the kinds of treatments to which it applies; might not be applied at all if your wishes regarding particular treatment in a specific circumstance are not known; and can fail because of physician and family concerns

The model document in Appendix B moderates some of the problems of living wills but cannot eliminate them. For that reason, if you want to be as sure as possible that your plans for avoiding life-sustaining treatment will work, you should also make a health-care durable power of attorney unless you do not know an appropriate agent.

CHAPTER 2

Understanding and Addressing Concerns of Your Providers, Family, and Agents

Withholding and withdrawing life-sustaining treatment often is troubling for all involved, but that does not have to be. This chapter will help you understand some of the basic concerns and address them constructively and effectively.

ISSUES

For Providers

Physicians often relate to disease differently than laypeople do. The medical way is to fight disease with every available means. Physicians base decisions on physical facts, which they see as objective—things that can be proved and measured—and may discount subjective things such as patients' feelings and goals. This approach can result in focusing on isolated body functions (a blood count, an electrolyte level, etc.), which can generate more and more treatment, because body functions can often be manipulated virtually to the moment of death.

Health-care planning documents con-flict with the medical approach, because they treat medical facts as less important than patients' values about health and life. As the American College of Physicians says in its ethics manual for physicians:

Because physicians invest so much in acquiring the necessary knowledge for making diagnostic and therapeutic decisions, it is often difficult for them to accept the fact that what is the "best" decision for a particular patient (in the opinion of the patient) may not be the "right" decision for that patient (in the opinion of the physician).

That statement can be true for nurses, too. As physicians focus on diagnosis and treatment, nurses are devoted to giving care. Sometimes nurses cannot accept the fact that patients may not want all that they offer. This can especially be a problem in long-term-care facilities, such as nursing homes and rehabilitation centers.

Physicians who accept patient decision making in principle may still have problems accepting health-care planning documents in practice, because desire to help patients and respect for patient choice can conflict.

Documents often do not answer treatment questions clearly. Even when they do, physicians may doubt that patients really could have known what quality of life or medical treatment they would find acceptable in the future. Physician doubts can be even sharper if agents say to stop ongoing treatments that patients had personally accepted when they could speak for themselves.

Often physicians cannot know for sure whether treatment will improve quality of life, or only sustain life, until after the treatment has been tried for some time. Depending on the circumstances, that can make providers feel that they should start or continue life-sustaining treatment.

Apart from conflict between physician judgment and patient choice, physicians almost always have trouble withholding or withdrawing life-sustaining treatment if a family member objects—even when physicians know what the patients would want. (Close relatives usually know when consideration is being given to withholding or withdrawing life-sustaining treatment based on a health-care planning document. In Arizona, Connecticut, Colorado, Nebraska, and Ohio, laws require physicians to notify certain family members.) Family opposition is a major reason health-care planning documents fail.

In principle, treatment decisions are up to patients. But in practice, if patients lose decision-making capacity (or even before then, especially if they are elderly) physicians often defer to family. Providers may see family members as the "natural" decision makers. Physicians may also feel that patients who have lost decision-making capacity (particularly those who are comatose) no longer have an interest in how they are treated, but that family members do, so family choices should prevail. (That view is short-sighted, both ethically and practically. A major factor in the morale of seriously ill people is their *expectation* about how they will be treated, including whether their personal choices about life and death will be respected. Anticipation that they will *not* be respected can cause intense suffering.) Whatever the reason, a physician may tend to act as if family members have become patients in place of the sick person, giving them effective veto power over the patient's intention to limit medical treatment.

These problems aside, some physicians and nurses feel that their knowledge and experience give them the right and the obligation to decide what care patients should have, and that those who seek their help implicitly consent to accept whatever they think is best. Other physicians and nurses may feel that the very nature of medicine and nursing is to give care, and that patients cannot reject the care that providers devote themselves to giving.

Finally, physicians may worry that following a health-care planning document will bring criticism from other providers or from a patient's family. That fear can be especially acute if a family member threatens legal action.

Part of what all this means is that you should choose a physician with whom you feel comfortable, who understands and accepts your intentions, and who will support your choices even in difficult circumstances. Don't be afraid to talk with a physician about these matters; the physician you want will welcome it.

For Family

Various stresses can make family members push for maximal life prolongation. If they are unsure about what their loved one would want, that uncertainty can make them request more treatment. They may feel that love and responsibility require "not giving up" and "doing everything possible." Sometimes family members will feel guilty about something in their relationship with a sick person, such as not having maintained close contact over the years, and may feel that continuing treatment somehow helps to make up for that. If certain family members would want maximal treatment for themselves, they may project their own wishes onto their relatives. Some relatives might feel that to stop life support would make them partly responsible for the death. One family member might feel pressure to go along with others who want maximum treatment, or that to stop treatment would disappoint or anger a physician or nurse. Finally, family members might just want to delay having to face their loved one's death.

For Agents

Most people who name an agent choose a family member, who may be subject to the influences addressed in the previous section. The kinds of stresses family members experience, however, often affect nonfamily agents as well.

TALKING AND LISTENING

What should you do to address these issues? It's very basic: talk about them, and listen to others' concerns.

With Your Agents

If you make a durable power of attorney for health care you need to talk with your prospective agents (don't neglect your alternate if you have one), preferably before meeting with your physician.

First, you need to determine if they are willing and feel able to serve as your agent. Love and respect for you are not enough. If a person has doubts about whether he will be able to deal with medical information, handle possible resistance from your family or physician, make decisions based on your values, or actually make a decision to stop life support, then for both his sake and yours he should not be your agent. Also, your agents need to talk with you for the same reason as your family and providers; hearing from you and having a chance for you to hear their concerns is vital to their peace of mind about your intentions. Don't ever name an agent without first talking to him. Consequences could range from unnecessary stress on him and on your family to your intentions failing entirely.

If an agent is willing and able to serve, then you need to explain your intentions to her to ensure that she understands what you want. Remember that she might have to decide questions that your power of attorney does not clearly answer.

Use your actual, completed (except for signatures) documents to guide discussion. Don't worry that you might change them in some way after you meet with your physician. Using your documents will help you be sure to cover everything, and will encourage your agents to ask "what if" questions. Also, the specificity of the model documents in this book can help agents understand just what is expected of them. Finally, discussing your documents will reinforce that if you ever become unable to speak for yourself and a question arises about what you would want, your documents are where to look for guidance.

If you have family members who do not know your agents, try to bring everyone together to talk. You don't want them to meet for the first time during a crisis. Also, a family conference that includes your agents can help your family realize that if you become unable to communicate your wishes personally then your agents will speak for you. Finally, group discussion can expose potential family-agent conflicts, and provide a setting for trying to resolve them.

If possible, take your agents (again, both primary and alternate if possible) with you when you meet with your physician. You are asking your physician to rely on one of them if you become unable to make decisions yourself. Your physician may feel more comfortable working with an agent she has met, and who has heard what you and she had to say.

With Your Health-Care Providers

Each provider and patient brings expectations and needs to a relationship. The more these overlap the more likely health-care planning documents are to work.

There are two reasons to talk with providers. The first is to find out whether you feel comfortable with the people (the physician, and sometimes a nursing director in a long-term-care facility) who would be in charge of your care. The second is to make sure that they understand and accept your choices about use of life-sustaining treatment, and if necessary feel able to defend them. Rarely will a physician feel able to advocate for your choices based on your documents alone, even if you have been a long-time patient. She may need the additional assurance that personal discussion can provide.

Your health-care planning documents are most likely to work if your physician has had a chance to see that you know and mean what your documents say, and that you heard what she had to say about your plans.

Don't avoid talking with your physician because you are afraid that he might see an issue differently than you do. Discussion can change minds (yours, your provider's, or both) and foster mutual respect. Also, if there is serious resistance or opposition, the earlier you know about it the easier you can deal with it.

Almost all physicians are very willing to talk, but you may have to take the first step. Make a special appointment (even if your insurance won't cover it). You want your physician to see that you take the matter seriously. Also, discussion tagged on to an appointment made for another purpose can end up being incomplete because of time constraints. Before the appointment send your physician a copy of your documents, completed except for signatures, with a note that you want to give her a chance to read them in advance. My clients have reported that discussions of their documents have taken anywhere from five minutes to two hours. (The longest time was for a person who had a complex disease, and met with a treatment team rather than a single physician.) Most people don't need to schedule a long appointment, but if one appointment doesn't give you enough time don't hesitate to make another.

Consider writing a list of things you want to discuss, including particular questions you might have. Compiling a list may help you think of things that would not occur to you on the spot in your doctor's office, or that might slip your mind then.

Wait to sign your documents until after

you meet with your physician, for these important reasons:

- You might hear something that changes your thinking. Information on which you have based your choices about life-sustaining treatment might be mistaken or incomplete, or might not apply to you because of your personal health condition. Medical diagnostic and treatment capabilities can change suddenly, so your information may not be current. (See comments on document renewal in Chapter 4.) Discussion with your physician might change your perspective on what you want in certain circumstances, and/or affect how you express your wishes in your documents.
- You want your physician to know that what she has to say is important to you. That concern comes across more effectively if you haven't signed the documents before you discuss them.
- Health-care planning documents are legal instruments, and many physicians resent legal intrusions into medical practice. Discussion before signing can "delegalize," so to speak, and personalize the process between you and your physician.

When your documents are in final form, ask your physician to promise to honor your wishes. Making a promise will not avoid the reluctance your physician might feel when he is confronted with actually withholding or stopping life-sustaining treatment; but the promise will become part of your physician's commitment to you. If your physician will not promise to withhold or stop life-sustaining treatment in the circumstances your documents describe, you need to know why. Then you need to decide whether you are running an unacceptable risk of your in-

tentions being overridden. If you think you are, you should consider changing physicians.

Some physicians are poor listeners. A physician who won't listen to you in person probably won't pay attention to your documents either. If you feel your physician thinks that what he says to you is more important than what you tell him, change physicians.

Don't be afraid to change physicians. Your doctor probably won't take it personally; no physician can suit every patient, and she'll want you to be served by someone with whom you feel comfortable. You don't have to discuss your reasons for changing if you don't want to, although if you ask your current physician for a referral to someone else she might ask you why. Your new physician can get a copy of your medical records directly from your previous doctor.

If you change physicians after making health-care planning documents, you should discuss your documents with your new doctor.

With Your Family

Family conflicts often complicate decision making in a health crisis, and family opposition can cause your intentions to fail. On the other hand, family support can confirm your intentions and choices. It is crucial that you discuss your intentions with your immediate family (spouse, adult children, parents, adult siblings), and give them a chance to share their concerns with you. This may not head off every problem, but giving everyone a chance to listen and be heard can do a lot to overcome resistance and build acceptance of your intentions. You might feel uncomfortable with the idea of discussing dying and death with your family, or you may be concerned that they will be uncomfortable. Once discussion starts, though, it usually goes surprisingly well.

Use your documents to guide discussion; again, that will help you cover everything, encourage people to talk, and reinforce the authority of your documents and your agents.

Think about whether to talk to your family members together, individually, or both. Group discussion can reduce the risk of people later having different recollections or understandings of what you said. Also, group conversation can bring out conflicts between family members over treatment issues or related matters that could be missed talking one-on-one.

Assure your family that to honor your choices is a loving and respectful act, and ask them to promise you that they will do so. If, after discussion, one or more immediate family members will not do that, you have a potentially serious problem that you need to address. You need to know what the problem is, and why. If you think someone else's support (your physician, clergy, another relative, etc.) might influence an objecting family member, by all means try to get them together. If the family member still can't accept your intentions, ask whether she could accept *others* honoring them as long as she is not asked to participate. Unless a problem is definitely resolved you need to explain the situation to your physician, and ask him to recommit to your intentions despite family opposition. If your physician will not do that, then you should consider changing physicians. You should also discuss potential family opposition with your agents.

Depending on the situation, you should consider discussing family opposition with a lawyer who is knowledgeable about medical decision making and health-care planning issues.

You should also consider stating in your document that a family member (identify him or her specifically, such as "my mother, Mary Smith") opposes this or that intention, but that you expect your providers to respect your decisions. For example, you could say (in the guardianship section of the power of attorney, which is discussed in Chapter 5):

If someone other than my agent is appointed as my guardian, I do not want my mother, Mary Smith, to be appointed. I am concerned that making decisions about use of life-sustaining treatment would be too stressful for her. I am also concerned that she would base such decisions on her sense of what she would want for herself, instead of on my intentions and choices.

You might wonder if you really need get into as much detail as the model documents do, and discuss your intentions and documents with your family, providers, and agents. You may feel your wishes are known and don't have to be spelled out, or that discussion will be uncomfortable or inconvenient. The reality is that even people who care about you and know you well probably *don't* know your wishes well enough; unless you talk with them and get their support, your intentions are at risk of failing.

In a way, health-care planning documents are like insurance: you can't know before a loss just how much protection you really need. Short but uninformative documents might work, but there is a real risk that they will not. Likewise, documents might work without discussion, but they are much more likely to work with it. Why accept significant risk that you can avoid? No document can be guaranteed to work, since so much depends on the people who are asked to accept them. But sound documents together with personal discussion can increase the likelihood that your intentions will be respected if your documents are ever needed.

CHAPTER 3

Questions and Answers

This chapter provides answers to the most common questions people have about health-care planning documents.

1. Who can make health-care planning documents?

Any mentally sound adult can make such a document, and sometimes certain minors. In most states the age of majority is 18. In Nebraska the minimum age for making health-care planning documents is 19.

If you are physically unable to complete a document, have someone else do that for you at your direction. (See Question 5, Part g.) In no state can another person make a health-care power of attorney for you except at your request. (In several states, however, if you do not have a health-care power of attorney then certain people [usually relatives] can direct your providers to withhold, withdraw, or continue life-sustaining treatment without direction from you.)

If you have reason to believe your mental status may be questioned, consult an attorney who is experienced with guardianships. Guardianship is a legal process in which a judge decides whether a person has become unable to manage personal or business affairs (see Chapter 5). For lawyer sources, see Question 5.

Minors who live on their own, are married, or are particularly mature and have strong religious or other personal beliefs regarding life-sustaining medical treatment in general, or about particular treatments such as blood transfusions, might be able to make valid health-care planning documents. There is legal support for that in Florida, Idaho, Illinois, Indiana, Maine, New Jersey, Pennsylvania, and Virginia. (Particular qualifications vary among those states.) In several other states the law does not authorize documents by minors but does not exclude them either. In most states, a minor who wants to make such documents needs to consult an attorney who is knowledgeable about health-care planning issues. Exceptions are Pennsylvania, if you are a high school graduate or are married, and Indiana, if you are married or in military service.

2. Who should make health-care planning documents?

Anyone who wants to avoid life-sustaining medical treatment in some circumstances should have health-care planning documents, because anyone can experience an illness or injury for which life-sustaining treatment might be used. Health-care planning is not only for people who are old or sick.

3. If I have family members or a physician I trust to make decisions for me if I become unable to make decisions personally, do I

really need health-care planning documents?

Yes, for three reasons.

First, asking or agreeing to stop, or not start, life-sustaining treatment can be very stressful for family members. Telling your loved ones what you want can lift the burden of decision from them, by helping them see that the decision to avoid life-sustaining treatment is yours, not theirs.

Second, without specific information from you, someone else's decision might not be the one you would have wanted. Research shows that family members and physicians are poor at predicting others' preferences for use of life-sustaining treatment, and that they often disagree with each other about how a patient would decide.

Third, in most states the legal authority of family members to make health-care decisions for each other is not clear. When a person is very sick physicians customarily look to family members for decisions. If everyone agrees about use of life-sustaining treatment there might not be a problem. But, if even one family member disagrees and there is any question about who has final authority or about what the patient would have wanted, then such treatment is likely to be used unless someone else is prepared to push hard for a different decision. Even when agreement is unanimous, sometimes physicians or health-care institutions are afraid to limit life-sustaining treatment in the face of uncertainty about who can make decisions. Such uncertainty can be avoided by a health-care power of attorney, and sometimes by a living will.

4. Should health care-planning documents be drafted by an attorney?

Attorney involvement is normally not necessary. The model documents in this book (or other forms that you might use) can be completed without attorney participation. Also, attorney involvement is usually not helpful. Most attorneys do not know enough about medical decision making—particularly about withholding and withdrawing life-sustaining treatment—to give advice. Few attorneys can do more than copy whatever document appears in your state's laws (these forms can be gotten at many stationery stores for about a dollar, and most appear in Appendix D) or in some other source. As of this writing most statutory forms standing alone are grossly inadequate; they are too vague for physicians, family, and agents to know what a patient would or would not want in many circumstances, and they understate legal rights.

When you are ready to make health-care planning documents you should consider checking whether the law in your state has changed in any important way since this book was finished (December 31, 1992). One way to do that is through an attorney, but you can get the most current information, at minimal cost, from Choice in Dying (formerly the Society for the Right to Die/Concern for Dying), 200 Varick Street, New York, NY 10014, telephone 212–366–5540. This organization is also the best source if you need information on more than one state, because most law offices only have the laws of their own state. Don't rely on information that health-care facilities distribute; it might not be current, specific, or complete.

5. When do I need to consult a lawyer, and how do I find one who is knowledgeable about health-care planning issues?

You need to consult a lawyer if:

a. You have a question about your rights, your providers' obligations, or the rights of others (family, agents, health-care providers, etc.) who you expect will be involved, or will want to be involved, in decisions about your health care, or if you have any other legal questions. No book is a substitute for personal legal advice.

b. You want to make a health-care planning document and you are a minor (except in Indiana and Pennsylvania as noted above).

c. A family member opposes your intentions regarding life-sustaining treatment.

d. Your current physician or facility (or, the physician or facility you expect will be your provider) will not accept your choices, and you cannot find a suitable provider who will; or, in the case of a facility, if another facility is available but you do not want to go there.

e. A legal action is started to appoint a guardian (or your state's equivalent) for you.

f. You think your mental capacity might be questioned when you sign your documents, or you have reason to believe that if your documents ever need to be implemented someone might claim you did not understand them when you made them.

g. You are physically unable to complete documents personally and your state law does not authorize someone else to do that for you at your direction. (Chapter 6, Tables 1 and 2, show which states authorize that.) Such laws should apply as well to other document contents that need to be supplied. If your state law does not authorize signature by others and you cannot complete your documents yourself, you should consider consulting a lawyer about how to proceed.

h. Your health-care planning documents, or those of a person for whom you are the agent, are resisted or opposed.

i. You want your health-care durable power of attorney to take effect—in other words, you want someone else to make your health-care decisions for you—while you still are able to make decisions for yourself. (First discuss this with your physician if you have one.)

j. You learn the law has changed in a way that is important to you and you have questions about whether or how to change your documents.

To find a knowledgeable lawyer, you can contact:

a. The lawyer referral service of your county bar association. Ask for referral to lawyers (get more than one name) who are experienced with planning for withholding and withdrawing life-sustaining medical treatment. If the service can't provide that (which in many places will be the case), request lawyers experienced with guardianship. Be aware that lawyer referral services do not screen for experience or expertise; usually any attorney licensed to practice in the state can sign up. A lawyer in any urban or large suburban county who seeks guardianship work and has practiced law at least five years should have had experience with health-care planning issues. Ask lawyers you call about their experience.

b. Various community groups that serve senior citizens or people with serious health impairments (for example, cancer support groups).

c. Organizations devoted to education and advocacy regarding certain serious illnesses such as AIDS, cancer, diabetes, and kidney disease.

d. State offices of the Hemlock Society.

6. Are there particular requirements for the contents of health-care planning documents?

Yes. Typical requirements are that a document state the maker's intentions, be dated and signed, and be witnessed by qualified witnesses and/or notarized by a notary public. Requirements for each state are listed in Chapter 6, Tables 1 and 2.

To ensure that documents are made voluntarily, most states exclude people who might have some personal interest in life-sustaining treatment being withheld or withdrawn from being witnesses or agents. The people most commonly excluded are close relatives, heirs, and health-care providers and their employees. Exclusions vary from state to state. Again, see Chapter 6, Tables 1 and 2.

7. If I refuse life-sustaining treatment, will I still be cared for?

Yes. Physicians and nurses are ethically obligated to continue caring for their patients even if some particular treatment (whether life-sustaining or not) is rejected. Ethically and legally, they can never abandon a patient. Particularly, comfort care must always be provided.

The law in many states allows providers to refuse to withhold or withdraw life-sustaining treatment for reasons of conscience (or in the case of a facility, based on its own policy, subject to some restrictions). Ethically, if a physician is not willing to implement a patient's rejection of treatment she should transfer responsibility for care to another physician who is willing (or if a patient has an agent, help the agent do that). This is based on the principles of respect for patients as individuals and the responsibility not to treat a patient without consent. Implicitly the same principles apply to facilities, although usually a physician rather than a facility is immediately responsible for a patient's care. The law favors transfer, too, if a physician or facility will not accept a patient's choice. State laws vary from making the physician responsible for arranging

transfer, to obligating him to help others make arrangements, to telling him only not to impede or unreasonably delay transfer.

A nurse who objects to participating in withholding or withdrawing life-sustaining treatment can ask the nursing supervisor for transfer from the case.

8. Can a physician or nurse, or a hospital, nursing home, or other health-care facility, or any other person or entity, require that I have a health-care planning document, or use a particular form of document, or revoke a document?

No. A federal law called the Patient Self-Determination Act prohibits all facilities that receive Medicare or Medicaid money (which nearly every facility does) from discriminating in admission or care because a person does or does not have a health-care planning document. That applies to document form and revocation, too. Many states have similar laws that apply to all health-care professionals and to all health-care facilities except federal (military and Veterans Administration) hospitals. Federal hospitals have or will have nondiscrimination policies consistent with the Patient Self-Determination Act.

9. When do health-care planning documents become effective?

The documents in this book apply when, because of illness or injury, a person who completes them becomes unable to make health-care decisions personally.

Making a health-care decision involves understanding medical and other information about treatment options (including foregoing treatment), making a decision, and communicating that decision. As long as you can do these things your health-care planning documents do not apply because you can make decisions yourself. To be valid your decision does not have to be what anyone else sees as best for you.

A person may be able to make certain decisions but not others, depending on the complexity of information involved. Also, decision-making ability can vary, even in short periods of time (such as over the course of a day).

Decision-making ability is more likely to be questioned when a person rejects medical advice than when he accepts it. It is also more likely to be questioned the more serious the consequences of a decision. A provider might accept a patient's refusal to stop smoking, for example, but challenge the patient's refusal to accept amputation of a gangrenous foot.

There is no objective "medical" test for determining whether a person can make a decision. Usually inability is apparent to physicians and laypeople alike. When it is not, ideally it should be determined by agreement among the patient's physicians, her agent if she has one, her family, and the patient herself if she can participate. (Often an attending physician will ask a psychologist, or another physician such as a neurologist or psychiatrist, to help assess decision-making ability.) The model durable power of attorney in this book provides for determination by agreement between the attending physician and agent, with the agent having the option of having a second physician determine the matter if the agent and the attending physician disagree. For living wills such decisions are up to physicians alone, or in some states physicians and psychologists. Decision-making ability will not be determined by a court unless an important treatment decision is being held up because of disagreement about who should make it or what it should be.

10. What if my wishes change? How do I change my health-care planning documents?

Your documents should always state your current wishes.

Don't rely on an oral understanding or agreement with a physician, or anyone else, that differs from what your documents say. Side-agreements invite conflict between the person with whom you have them and others who believe you want what your documents say. Even when everyone concerned knows about a separate understanding, later on they might remember it differently. And, if an understanding is with a certain physician, he might not be the one in charge of your care if your documents ever come into play.

If the models in this book say something that is not true for you, or do not include something that is important to you, then you should change them. Delete material by drawing a line through anything you don't want. Add material on the lines provided in the forms for that purpose, or attach an additional page.

If you delete material or add comments, you need to initial and date the line-out or addition and have your witnesses, and a notary public if you use one, do the same. (Any page you add should be signed, not just initialed.) These measures verify that each deletion or addition was made by you, when the document was executed.

If you want to change a health-care planning document after it has been signed, witnessed, and notarized (other than changing the address or telephone number of an agent in a durable power of attorney), it is best to make a whole new document.

Note that in Vermont a health-care durable power of attorney cannot be changed in any way; the entire document must be reexecuted.

Don't forego making an important change for want of a notary, or even qualified witnesses. Even if a change is not formally legal, your physician (and a judge in court) should honor it as an expression of your intentions.

Note: If you make both a living will and a health-care power of attorney, and later your wishes change, be sure to change both documents, not just one of them (unless you decide to revoke one document entirely—for example, if you decide not to have a power of attorney any longer).

11. If the law changes after I make a document, will my document still be valid?

Almost certainly. Typically when new laws are enacted or existing laws are amended, the new law or amendment validates existing documents.

It is not likely that a new law or amendment would narrow previous rights. If it did so, your entire document would not become invalid; instead, any part of it that was no longer legal simply would not be legally enforceable. A legally unenforceable provision should still be honored by your physician, out of respect for you, unless the law expressly prohibits your choice.

Sometimes legal changes expand or clarify rights. The model documents in this book include language intended to automatically incorporate new rights.

Sometimes documents made after a law changes must include some particular language or be in a certain form. This is another reason to consider checking whether your state's law has changed since December 31, 1992. You can find that out by calling or writing Choice in Dying, in New York City. (They can tell you whether a state's law has changed, and if so they might be able to give you some information about whether the change imposes any requirements for documents. For further information, you can contact a lawyer or a senior citizens legal aid or health advocacy group.)

12. Are documents I make in my home state legal in other states or other countries?

Generally, documents that are legal in one state are legal in other states. Certain provisions, however, might not be accepted by providers, or be legally enforceable, if the law of the state where implementation is sought does not authorize them or if it prohibits them.

You should not expect health-care planning documents made in the United States to be honored in other countries, although they might be. Talk with a trustworthy doctor or lawyer there for advice.

13. Should I have both a directive or declaration and a durable power of attorney?

Yes. It would be possible to make a single health-care planning document that would serve as both a power of attorney and a living will, and laws in a few states offer such combined forms. These forms, however, tend to do a poor job of informing people about their health-care planning rights, helping people decide what they want, and communicating their intentions. In most states, there are separate living will and health-care power of attorney laws, often with significantly different provisions. Until separate laws are consolidated, or at least harmonized, separate documents are advisable.

Some states that authorize living wills do not yet have laws that expressly authorize durable powers of attorney for health care. If a provider will not accept an agent's authority in these states, then a directive or declaration can be important insurance. Where there are health-care power of attorney laws, a directive or declaration also can serve as important backup if an agent is unavailable when a decision needs to be made.

14. Should I make a durable power of attorney for health care if my state has not yet authorized them?

Yes.

A health-care durable power of attorney might be legally valid under a general durable power of attorney law. Also, more states are passing laws specifically authorizing health-care powers of attorney, and new laws usually validate existing documents. Further, if you were to become unable to make health-care decisions when you happen to be in another state that does have an applicable law, your document may be accepted there. If necessary it might be possible for your agent to move you to such a state.

Apart from legal authority, a well-drafted document can be morally persuasive with your physician and family. (The same is true for directives and declarations in the few states whose laws do not recognize them.) A durable power of attorney would probably be admissible as evidence of your wishes in legal proceedings in which providing, withholding, or withdrawing treatment is an issue.

15. Who should I choose as my agent?

The people you choose as your agent and alternate agent need to:

• *Know you well.* Health-care planning documents cannot anticipate every circumstance that might occur; your agents need to know how you feel and what you think about life-sustaining treatment and other treatment issues.

• *Be able to separate their own values and choices from yours.* Your agent is supposed to base her decisions for you on *your* intentions. Only if she does not know what you would want should she decide as she personally believes is in your best interest. So, she needs to be able to separate her values and choices from yours and decide as you would want. Some people just cannot do that. That kind of person should not be your agent, unless you feel confident that her values and yours are the same.

• *Be able to ask physicians questions, and understand medical information that can be complex, conflicting, and shaded to steer him to a particular decision.* Information about diagnosis and prognosis, and risks and benefits of various treatment options, can be involved. There can be a lot of facts and choices to think through. Ideally a physician helps an agent decide what to do, by talking about the agent's concerns and providing needed information, including things the agent might not think to ask, or be afraid to ask. Unfortunately that doesn't always happen. In that case, an agent needs to ask for what he needs.

• *Be able to make decisions, perhaps under great stress.* Some people cannot bring themselves to make painful decisions, especially if someone else (particularly someone with apparent authority, such as a physician) disagrees with them. They may delay decisions, or defer to others. You shouldn't put that kind of person in the position of making decisions for you about life-sustaining treatment.

• *Be able to push for action on decisions if necessary.* Deciding is one thing, doing is another. Your agent might have to overcome resistance or opposition to accomplish your wishes, or to do what's best for you if your wishes are not known. Summoning the certitude and emotional strength to do that can be very difficult (especially if your agent doesn't know you well). Your agent needs to be able to push her decision. That might mean requesting a care conference with the whole treatment team, if there is one; meeting with a facility administrator, medical and nursing directors, and ethics committee if there is one; changing physicians; transfering you to another facility or to someone's home; or, as a last resort, going to court.

• *Be someone you trust completely.* Some powers of attorney limit agents' authority. The model power of attorney in this book does not do that, for two reasons. First, limitations might prevent your agent from acting for you in circumstances you haven't foreseen. If you limit his authority you might inadvertently exclude options you would want him to consider. Second, limiting authority sends conflicting messages to health-care providers. Instead of saying that you want them to rely completely on your agent, it says "I trust my agent, but only so far." If you express limited trust, your providers and family might, too.

If you feel you want to limit your agent's authority, think again about your choice of agent. If you do not trust a person to make certain foreseeable decisions, then she might not be the right person to make unforeseeable ones for you, either.

Most people choose a relative to be their agent, and for many people that is a good choice. But, from the considerations just discussed you can see that sometimes the best choice will be someone else. An agent's effectiveness can mean the difference between your health-care durable power of attorney working or failing. So, careful consideration in choosing your agent is just as important as what you say in your document.

The model durable power of attorney lets you name an alternate in addition to your primary agent. You do not have to name an alternate; if an appropriate person is not available, don't name someone just because the form has a space for that. (Cross out the space if you don't use it.)

If you know two people who would be equally good agents, and one lives nearby but the other at a great distance, consider naming the one closer to you as your agent and the other as your alternate. If your agent were needed and lived at a distance, she would have to travel to you or try to function by telephone, making an already trying situation even tougher. Having to make troubling decisions a long way from home can be hard emotionally. Also, an agent can be needed over a longer period of time than she can be away from her family, job, and other responsibilities. Trying to function as an agent by telephone can also be difficult. Information can be hard to get and discuss adequately; emotional stresses can be intensified if the agent feels torn between responsibilities at home and a sense of duty to be with you; and trust between agent and physician can also be harder to establish over the telephone.

In many states the law excludes certain people from acting as agents (see Chapter 6, Table 1). Be sure not to name an excluded person as your agent or alternate; that could cause your document to be rejected.

If the person you would like as your agent is excluded by your state's law, you can say in your durable power of attorney that you want the agent you name to consult with the excluded person. If you do that you should explain your reason. For example, for someone disqualified because she is employed by your health-care provider, you could say:

For any decision about whether to start or to stop life-sustaining treatment, I want my agent to consult my sister-in-law, Susan Smith, M.D. Dr. Smith and I know each other well, and I trust and value her judgment. I have not made her my agent because she is disqualified by law as an employee of my health-care provider.

Sometimes people want to name joint agents. Think carefully before you do that. When multiple decision makers are involved, confusion and misunderstanding can occur among them, and with providers. If joint agents cannot reach agreement, then one dissenter in effect has veto power over the other(s). Decision making can be delayed if all joint agents are not available when needed. If you want family members to talk together about what to do, by all means tell them so. But give just one of them authority.

Note that in Illinois naming joint agency is not legally permissible.

16. Should durable powers of attorney for health care, and for financial matters, be combined in one document?

No.

The most important reason is that the same person might not be the best decision maker for both health care and finances. An agent for financial matters might not need any of the attributes of a health-care agent, and a person who would be a good health-

care agent might not know how to manage financial affairs.

There is also the matter of privacy; there is no reason for strangers to know more than necessary about your personal affairs. Your health-care providers do not need to know your financial interests and plans, and your bank and insurance company do not need to know your intentions for health care.

In California and Florida the law requires that powers of attorney for health-care and other purposes be separate.

17. Can health-care planning documents be revoked?

Yes. In most states they can be revoked at any time, by any act that communicates that intention (such as an oral or written statement, or tearing up a document).

Execution of a new health-care planning document usually revokes other such documents you may have made previously.

Warning: Many health-care facilities offer health-care planning forms to new patients on admission. These forms are often very restrictive, in ways that might not be apparent to you at the time, and often give inadequate guidance for decision making. If you complete such a form, you might automatically revoke a prior document that states your intentions more fully and more accurately. So, if you already have a health-care planning document that expresses your wishes, do not sign another form at a health-care facility. Tell the facility you already have a document or documents, and provide copies.

If you revoke a document, retrieve the original and all copies if you can (except as described in the next paragraph). If a health-care provider will not return a document (some providers will not remove anything from a patient record), and you have made a new document, give the provider the new document; the more recent date on the new document should effectively revoke the older document. If you want to revoke but not replace a document, give the provider a written notice of revocation to put in your record. (See Appendix C, except for Mississippi; for that state, see Appendix D.)

Be sure to keep the original or a copy of each health-care planning document you ever make. Also, have your agent (or if you don't have one, then another trusted person, such as a family member or lawyer) keep a copy of every document. Sometimes questions arise concerning the course of a person's health-care values and choices over time. Past documents can be important evidence.

In New York and Mississippi, the laws say a person must be competent to revoke a health-care planning document. However, medically appropriate life-sustaining treatment will not be withheld or withdrawn from a person who says he wants it even if he is incompetent.

Note that in Mississippi, revocation of a power of attorney must be in writing. Revocation of a directive also must be written, unless the person who wishes to revoke is physically unable to write, in which case revocation can be oral. Written revocation of a directive must be in a form that appears in the law, and must be filed with the "bureau of vital statistics of the state board of health."

In several states (Florida, Kansas, Pennsylvania, Texas, Vermont, Washington, Wisconsin, and Wyoming), appointment of a guardian automatically revokes documents, or a guardian has legal authority to revoke a document.

In South Carolina the living will form in the law (see Appendix D, p. 208) has a section titled "APPOINTMENT OF AGENT (OPTIONAL)" in which you can name someone to revoke that document. If you do not want anyone to be able to revoke it, draw an X over all of block 1 in the form.

18. Does having or not having a health-care planning document affect eligibility for any kind of insurance? And, does stopping, or not starting, life-sustaining treatment affect insurance entitlements, such as health insurance or life insurance?

No. Federal law, and many state laws, prohibit any kind of discrimination related to health-care planning documents.

19. Legally, is withholding or withdrawing life-sustaining medical treatment as directed by a health-care planning document considered murder, suicide, or mercy killing anywhere in the United States?

No. Legally, the cause of death following stopping, or not starting, life-sustaining treatment is the health condition that prevented life from continuing without life support.

20. What if I don't understand something in the model Durable Power of Attorney for Health-Care Decisions, or in the Supplement to Directive or Declaration to Physicians?

Read the explanation of the provision in Chapter 5, pages 35–67. If you still have questions, talk to a physician you trust or to someone else who is knowledgeable about health-care matters. You should never include something in your document that you don't understand.

CHAPTER 4

How to Use the Model Documents

The model health-care planning documents we will discuss appear in two forms. The first form is a complete "Durable Power of Attorney for Health-Care Decisions" (see Appendix A). It is ready to use for most states. For a few states (noted in Chapter 6, Table 1) it must be used with a form or forms that appear in the state's law, and the state form may need to be completed in a certain way to coordinate with the model document. Coordination is very easy; instructions are in Appendix E. State forms you may need are in Appendix D, in alphabetical order by state.

The second form is a "Supplement to Directive or Declaration to Physicians" (see Appendix B). The supplement is basically the same as the power of attorney, but with the parts that apply only to agents omitted. The supplement is designed to be attached to the form of living will that appears in the law of each state that has one (see Appendix D) to make a complete document. In the few states where the living will law does not include a form (Delaware, New Jersey, New Mexico, and Ohio), or where there is no living will law at all (Massachusetts, Michigan, and New York), the supplement can be used as a complete, free-standing document, with very minor modifications that will be explained later.

In many states the forms in living will laws must be used; in other states the laws offer forms only as examples. It is wise to use your state form (if your state has one), even when it is optional and a poor guidance document. Providers (and their attorneys) are often more comfortable accepting a document that includes familiar material. That consideration is less important for state durable power of attorney forms because powers of attorney operate through agents, instead of standing alone as living wills must be able to do.

Everywhere—even in states where particular power of attorney or living will forms are required—additional statements of personal information and intentions can be added. Such statements have legal value, and should carry moral weight with health-care providers.

Again, your documents need to: (1) explain your wishes fully and clearly, to both health-care providers and laypeople; (2) bring out for discussion in advance issues that can be sticking points for providers, family, and agents; and (3) address legal requirements and gray areas. To do that, follow these steps:

1. Read through the model documents, but don't make any marks on them.

2. Read the section-by-section comments in Chapter 5.

These comments will help you understand the choices both model documents offer, decide and express what you want, and talk with your health-care providers, family, and agents to build commitment to respect your intentions.

3. Complete the documents, except for signatures and dates.

Follow the instructions in the documents. Do not leave any space blank. Every space in your completed documents should have something in it: your initials (to adopt a statement or option), a dash (to reject a statement or option), your written additional comments in spaces provided for them, or an X across any comment space you do not use. (This also applies to any form you use from Appendix D.)

4. If you make a durable power of attorney, talk with your intended agents.

Again, talking with your agents before finalizing your power of attorney is important to make sure they understand your wishes and an agent's responsibilities, and feel willing and able to carry them out.

5. Meet with a physician (preferably one whom you know, and who knows you) to discuss your documents.

Talking with a physician is important to make sure your choices are based on accurate medical information, and to get his understanding, acceptance, and support.

6. Discuss your documents with immediate family members, even if you are not close to them.

Even if a patient has a health-care planning document, most physicians will still consult family members about major treatment decisions. If even one opposes limiting life-sustaining treatment, many physicians will continue such treatment until disagreement is resolved or until the patient dies. Be sure to talk with your family.

7. Before you finalize a document, consider checking whether the law in any state of concern to you has changed in any important way since December 31, 1992.

The law of health-care planning documents is still new as law goes. New laws are being enacted and existing laws amended, and courts sometimes issue decisions that affect health-care planning rights. Such changes can occur at any time.

Again, a change probably would not invalidate an existing document, but a new document might have to satisfy some new requirement.

8. When you are completely satisfied with your documents, gather your witnesses, and a notary public if you use one, for signing and dating.

Make sure your agents and witnesses are not barred by any legal exclusion (see Chapter 6, Tables 1 and 2). Have them sign or initial, and date, all additions and deletions besides signing the witness statement at the end of a document.

Follow these steps to finalize your documents.

For directives and declarations: If a directive, declaration, or living will form for your state appears in Appendix D, complete it (noting any instructions for your state in Appendix E); complete the Supplement to Directive or Declaration to Physicians (Appendix B); staple the state form on top of the supplement, then sign and date both documents in the presence of your witnesses and/or notary public and have the documents witnessed and/or notarized as directed in Chapter 6, Table 2. (If feasible have them both witnessed and notarized, even if your state does not require both.)

If Appendix D does not include a living will form for your state, complete the supplement and have it witnessed and notarized. Cross out the words "Supplement to" in the document title, and each place it appears in the Statement of Witnesses and notary statement. You, your witnesses, and the notary should initial each of the crossouts.

For health-care powers of attorney: If a power of attorney form for your state appears in Appendix D, complete that form (noting any instructions for your state in Appendix E); complete the model Durable Power of Attorney for Health-Care Decisions (Appendix A); staple the various documents together, in this order: the "notice" or "warning" statement for Mississippi, Ohio, or Tennessee, or the "addendum" for Indiana (see Appendix D), then any state power of attorney form from Appendix D, then the model document; then sign and date each document in the presence of your witnesses and/or notary public and have the documents witnessed and/or notarized as directed in Chapter 6, Table 2. (Again, if feasible have each document both witnessed and notarized.)

If you make both a power of attorney and a living will for Arizona, see the special instruction in Appendix E.

In Michigan, North Dakota, and Oregon an agent must accept appointment in writing before he can act on your behalf. An acceptance statement is included in the Oregon and North Dakota power of attorney forms (which must be used in those states)

in Appendix D. A separate form for Michigan appears in Appendix D. An acceptance need not be signed at the same time as the power of attorney, but whether it is or is not, it should be part of the original power of attorney that you give to your agent, and the copy that you give to your alternate agent.

After completing your documents, do the following:

9. *Distribute them.*

Providers cannot honor documents they don't know exist, or haven't seen. Often relatives know a living will has been made but don't know where it is. Similarly, a person in a distant city may say he is a health-care agent, but if the provider has not seen the power of attorney document he cannot know that the person in fact is the agent, or what authority the agent has. To avoid those problems you need to be sure your documents get into the right hands.

Directive or declaration: If you have a personal physician, give her the original to put in your medical records. If you are in a health-care facility, give the facility a copy as well. If you live in a nursing home and do not have a personal physician, have the original put in your records. If you do not have a personal physician and are not in a facility, give the original to the person who is most likely to be called if you ever have a health emergency.

Additional copies of your directive or declaration should go to: (1) your agents if you have a durable power of attorney for health care; (2) close family members and close friends whom you believe your physicians might consult; and (3) your attorney if you have one.

Durable power of attorney for health-care decisions: Give the original to your agent. Give a copy to your alternate agent, if you have one, and to the same people and facilities that should receive your directive or declaration.

If you anticipate that you might become a patient at a certain hospital, and you have been a patient there before, ask that copies of both of your documents (if you make both) be put in your record. Some facilities accept documents from people who are not current patients; others do not.

Usually when patients are transferred between nursing homes and hospitals, or between hospitals, only brief summary records accompany them; health-care planning documents may be omitted. You should discuss with your present physician or other provider how you can ensure that your documents would follow you if you were transferred.

10. If you anticipate that you might enter a particular hospital or other facility, get a copy of the facility's written policies regarding withholding and withdrawing life-sustaining treatment.

The Patient Self-Determination Act requires almost all hospitals, nursing homes, hospices, home-care services, and prepaid medical plans such as health maintenance organizations to meet certain requirements concerning health-care planning. These include having written policies concerning directives and durable powers of attorney for health care. (Other requirements include giving every patient or resident, or member of a prepaid health plan, written information about rights under state law to refuse unwanted treatment, choose some kinds of treatment but not others, and make health-

care planning documents; ask and document whether a patient or resident has made health-care planning documents; ensure compliance with state laws concerning decision making about life-sustaining treatment; educate staff on applicable laws; and not discriminate against a patient or resident for having made, or not made, health-care planning documents.) Also, accredited hospitals are required to have written policies regarding use of cardiopulmonary resuscitation, and many have written policies about use of life-sustaining treatment generally. So, a facility should have some kind of policy for you to see.

Be aware that the Patient Self-Determination Act only requires facilities to tell you what choices your state laws allow you to make; it does not require that facilities or physicians implement your choices (but state law may do so). In fact, many facilities have certain restrictions. Nursing homes, particularly, may not permit withholding or withdrawing any life-sustaining treatment, or may permit withholding but not withdrawing treatment, or may apply special restrictions to artificial nutrition and hydration.

If a hospital or other facility you are considering says it does not have written policies on use of life-sustaining treatments and health-care planning documents, or will not give them to you when you request them, or if any policy is deficient in terms of openness to your choices, then you should choose another provider.

If only one facility is available and its policy is unacceptable to you, talk with your physician about whether the policy can be avoided in some way. If avoidance is impractical, request a meeting with the facility administrator, medical director, nursing director if the facility is an extended care facility, facility ethics committee (if there is one), and your physician, to see whether a mutually acceptable compromise, or an exemption, can be reached. If that fails, consider a facility in another locale; usually it is harder to fight than switch. If you are already a patient or resident in a facility and to transfer elsewhere is too burdensome, or if the facility did not tell you its policy when it received your documents and you just don't want to move, a court might order the facility to accept your intentions. If this becomes an issue for you, consult an attorney knowledgeable about patient rights issues.

11. You should renew your documents yearly, or sooner if there is a major change in your health status such as diagnosis of a life-threatening condition or admission to a nursing home or hospice.

No state requires renewal annually, or ever (except in Oregon, where powers of attorney expire after seven years unless the document maker is incapacitated then). But if, when a treatment question arises, a long time has passed since a document was made, questions sometimes arise about whether the document reflects current wishes. Annual renewal helps avoid such doubt. Also, renewal shows your concern about health-care planning issues over time,

which can make your current choices more persuasive.

You should definitely renew your documents if you experience a life-threatening illness. Providers sometimes question how much thought and information went into documents made when a person was healthy. Documents renewed after a person learns he has a serious health condition may be more persuasive. (In Utah, living wills can also have greater legal effect if they are made or renewed after a physician tells a patient he has a terminal condition.)

You should discuss documents with your physician yearly, too. This discussion will remind her to tell you about any new medical developments that might affect your choices. Also, you need to tell her if your intentions have changed in some way. Even if your choices remain the same, repeating intentions over time can help them sink in. (That goes for families and agents, too.)

Let your agent and family members know when you renew your documents, give them the latest documents, retrieve old versions (except from the one person who should keep a complete set), and alert them to any changes from earlier versions.

Finally, annual renewal is a reminder to check whether your documents should be amended to reflect any changes in the law that might have occurred since the documents were written or last renewed.

CHAPTER 5

Section-by-Section Instructions and Comments

This chapter takes you section by section through the model documents that appear in Appendixes A and B. The discussion focuses on the power of attorney (Appendix A), but applies equally to the same provisions in the supplement (Appendix B).

Print your name on the line below the document title. If you are physically unable to do that, and to do the initialing, signing, and dating that document preparation requires, see Chapter 6, Tables 1 and 2, for whether your state authorizes document completion by someone else. If it does not, and you are in a health-care facility, ask them how to proceed. If necessary, contact an attorney.

Power of attorney at 1 (Supplement at 1), "When I want this power of attorney to be effective." The power of attorney is in effect during any time when, because of illness or injury, you are unable to make your own health-care decisions. It emphasizes that you want to make your own health-care decisions when you can, and that even if you are unable to make some particular decision at a certain time you want to make others if you can.

It might be legal, at least in some states, to write a health-care planning document to be effective when you are still able to make decisions yourself but want someone else to do so for you. The model documents in this book do not do that, and no conscientious physician would withhold or withdraw life-sustaining treatment in reliance on a document or an agent when you can decide for yourself. If you think you would want someone else to make decisions for you even when you remain able to do so personally, you need to discuss your reasons with your physician, and perhaps consult an attorney who is experienced with health-care planning in your state.

This section also covers who should determine whether you cannot make a decision, and how uncertainty about that can be resolved. Many people just assume their physician will determine whether or not they are able to make decisions, and feel comfortable with that because they trust their physician, and/or because they assume that determining decision-making ability is a matter of medical expertise. But, many people come under the care of physicians who don't know them. And in fact, there is no objective medical test for decision-making ability; physicians form opinions about it based mainly on experience. Often the situation is clear; a person who is unconscious, for example, or severely demented, or heavily sedated, cannot make decisions. But sometimes circumstances are less clear. Then a physician's impression can be clouded by personal beliefs or feelings, including about the consequences of his capacity determination. If a physician feels that life-sustaining treatment should be continued but a patient's agent disagrees, and the physician believes he can get some kind of assent from the patient, that might influence the physician to conclude that the patient retains decision-making capacity; then the agent cannot make decisions.

It is important that a health-care durable power of attorney provide a mechanism for an agent to question a physician's opinion about capacity. The mechanism provided here is resolution by a consulting physician. (The supplement does not address resolution of uncertainty about decision-making capacity, because unless a patient has an agent—or possibly another surrogate decision maker under his state's law—that responsibility is the physician's.)

You need to know that in most states the law directs that incapacity be determined by the attending physician and another physician. In other words, the attending physician's agreement may be required. Most physicians will agree to consultation, and will consider a consultant's opinion. If your attending physician refuses to allow examination by a doctor your agent chooses, or insists that you have capacity when your agent and a consulting doctor do not, then your agent should request help (from a hospital ethics committee, for example) to change the attending physician's mind, or he should consider changing attending physicians.

In Michigan, New Hampshire, North

Carolina, and Oklahoma, the law allows people who object on religious grounds to being examined by a physician to have incapacity determined by someone else of their choosing. (That person cannot be: the agent or the document maker's health-care provider [North Carolina]; the agent or anyone ineligible to be the agent [New Hampshire]; the agent [Oklahoma]. In Michigan there is no restriction.) If that is your belief (and even if you do not live in one of those four states), you must write that in your document and write in the name of the person you would want to determine your incapacity. You can do that in the space at the end of Section 6 of the model power of attorney, Section 2 of the supplement, or on an additional page.

This section asks your physicians and agent to talk with you about your condition even if you are incapacitated. Many people want that; some do not. If you do not, draw a line through each line of the paragraph.

When decision-making ability has been lost it can sometimes be restored, at least temporarily. Trying to restore capacity can require trading one goal for another, such as giving less pain medication to reduce the sedation that potent pain medication can cause. At other times capacity can be improved without tradeoffs, by changing treatments. If you would want your physician or agent to try to restore lost capacity, you can indicate that by initialing the first space in "Temporary use of life-sustaining treatment" (Section 7 E in the power of attorney; Section 3 E in the supplement).

Some people assume that health-care planning documents apply to stopping, and not starting, life-sustaining treatment only in the event of a terminal condition. That is not true of the model documents in this book; they focus on quality of life, not expected length of life. (Shortcomings of "terminal condition" as a reason for limiting use of life-sustaining treatments are discussed later in this chapter.) It is important for all concerned to know that. That is the reason for the fifth paragraph in Section 1.

If a person has both a health-care power of attorney and a living will, there can be uncertainty about which document has priority. This can be important, even if both documents express the same intentions, because of the limitations in many state laws that might restrict choices that can be made based on a living will but not a power of attorney. Also, as explained above, powers of attorney are better means for securing health-care choices. For those reasons, the model documents provide that if you make both a power of attorney and a living will, you want the power of attorney to apply whenever possible.

Most state forms of living will say something to the effect that you intend that document to be the final expression of your wishes. That statement is not correct if in addition to the state form you execute a health-care power of attorney and/or the supplement. If you make a power of attorney or the supplement, be sure to cross out any "final expression" language in the state form.

The last paragraph of Section 1 allows you to authorize your agent to consent to autopsy, organ donation, donation of your body for medical research, and disposition of your remains. Historically, powers of attorney end at death. In some states (California, Georgia, Idaho, Illinois, Indiana, Kansas, Mississippi, Missouri, North Carolina, Tennessee, West Virginia, and Wyoming),

the law provides that they continue in effect for organ donation, and for autopsy and/or disposition of remains, either automatically or with your authorization. In other states the laws are silent. Whatever the law, health-care providers will usually accept an agent's consent after death if the patient's family does not object. If you anticipate objection from a family member, be sure to discuss that with all of your immediate family, your physician, and your agents.

If the law in your state is not clear about whether a durable power of attorney continues in effect after death, your agent should make arrangements for postdeath events before death occurs, if possible. Be sure to talk with your agent about this.

Like powers of attorney, directives and declarations usually terminate at death. But again, providers might honor your documented authorization for organ donation, autopsy, and research donation if no one objects.

Power of attorney at 2 and 3, Designation of health-care agent and alternate. Print the name of your agent and alternate, and their addresses and telephone numbers. It is important that you keep this information complete and up-to-date, because the document cannot work if your health-care provider cannot find an agent. If you don't know an appropriate alternate, don't name one; put an X across the blank space.

Power of attorney at 4, "The authority I want my agent to have." This part has two purposes. The first is to address a legal problem about whether your choices are limited by restrictions in state laws that authorize health-care planning documents. If your documents end up in court, the assertion that you do not intend limitations to be read into them, but rather that you claim your complete rights to provide for your health care, will give a judge sound grounds to enforce your intentions.

The second purpose is to give your agent the particular powers she needs to do what you are asking of her. These powers should be specified in the document. The reasons for them are as follows:

a. Consenting and refusing consent to any medical procedure; and withdrawing consent to any procedure already in use, even if started at your request or with your consent. This is an agent's most important power, because the main reason most people make health-care planning documents is to avoid unwanted treatment. Legally, treatment cannot be started without consent, and cannot be continued if consent is withdrawn. This statement means that if you become unable to make health-care decisions, your agent is the person who has authority to give consent, refuse consent, or withdraw consent for you.

b. Requesting particular medical procedures. Only rarely will an agent be in the position of requesting testing or treatment that a physician does not propose, but it does happen. Physicians are not required to accept an agent's (or patient's) request for particular testing or treatment. They are usually willing to discuss such matters, though, and usually end up either agreeing to the request or convincing the agent that it is inappropriate. If agreement cannot be reached, the agent can consider changing physicians and/or facilities.

c. Complete access to your medical records and information, including disclosure to others. Information about a patient is confidential; this part gives your provider permission to release it to your agent and to anyone else your agent directs.

Your agent needs access to information to make informed decisions about your health care. Information may also be needed by insurers (health, disability, life, and others) and other health-care providers. Information often needs to be shared so that a particular hospital, nursing home, or hospice can determine whether it would be an appropriate setting for a patient who is going to be transferred from another facility.

d. Employing and dismissing health-care providers (binding you, or any insurer of yours, to pay for the same). A physician who becomes involved in your case might not be willing to accept your intentions or choices, or might disagree with your agent about what you would want in particular circumstances. A facility might refuse to accept your agent's decision or your physician's order. If a disagreement is important enough and cannot be worked out, your agent needs authority to change providers.

This part also gives your agent permission to incur health-care costs chargeable to you and/or your insurer. If you have health insurance, Medicare, or Medicaid, whether any of those actually will be responsible for agent-incurred costs depends on what your insurance policy or federal and/or state law provides.

You need to be aware that insurance policies sometimes contain restrictions or exclusions that are invalid in some states. Also, insurance companies sometimes apply valid provisions improperly. If an insurer refuses to pay charges of a health-care provider (either a physician or a facility) hired by an agent, the agent should consult the state insurance commissioner, then if necessary an attorney knowledgeable about insurance coverage issues.

e. Removing you from any health-care

facility, even against medical advice, and transferring you to another facility or to a private residence or some other place. This part gives your agent authority to remove you from a health-care facility if she thinks that is best. Health-care facilities can be unsatisfactory in various respects, making transfer to another facility, or to a private home, desirable or necessary.

Often even seriously ill people can be cared for at home. Skilled home-care nursing services are widely available. The cost may be covered by private insurance or governmental sources (Medicare, Medicaid, Social Security, welfare, etc.).

f. Taking any other action necessary to do what you authorize in this document. Your agent might need some authority you do not foresee. If so, this part tries to provide it.

Sometimes health-care providers fear that if life-sustaining treatment is withheld or withdrawn they might be sued. To protect themselves they may request a release or waiver of liability. Providers have no right to refuse to withhold or withdraw treatment until they get a release or waiver. If a provider insists, no harm is done by giving one—but for the withholding or withdrawal of treatment only. An agent needs to be very careful about signing a general release or waiver, or a release or waiver that mentions negligence. If a release or waiver is demanded, your agent should get advice from an attorney knowledgeable about medical-legal issues.

Power of attorney at 5, "How I want my agent to make decisions for me." Sometimes health-care agents mistakenly think they should make decisions based on what they would want for themselves, or on what a physician or nurse says is best. Section 5 tells your agent to decide as he believes *you* would want.

Providers who are open to working with an agent can help her make good decisions, and you should encourage your agent to talk with them as advisors. But, impress on her that you want *her* to be the final decision maker.

Power of attorney at 6 (Supplement at 2), "Why I am making this power of attorney." A values statement explains the reasons for the choices you make later in the document about life-sustaining treatment. A thoughtful values statement emphasizes your seriousness in making your documents, and can make people more willing to believe that you mean what you say, which can help them accept your choices. Also, explaining your values makes it harder for others to substitute *their* values for yours. Finally, stating your values clearly and directly makes it harder for others to argue later that you would change your mind if you knew the particular circumstances that had come about. You are entitled to change your mind; but others should not presume you would have, as a way of avoiding your intentions.

It is important that the values statement be true for you. If something in it is not, delete it. If something else important to you is not there, add it in the space provided. If you make changes, keep in mind what the section needs to do: explain your basic values about health care, especially life-sustaining treatment; explain that you want your agent to make health-care decisions for you; and ask others to accept your agent's decisions as your own.

These are the basic values that limit use of life-sustaining treatment as expressed in the model document:

1. *Quality of life is more important than continuation of life.* The model documents

say that to you, quality of life is more important than length of life, and the quality of your life should be measured by your values.

2. *From the standpoint of quality of life, there is no difference between not starting a treatment in the first place and stopping treatment already in use.* You are entitled to say no to treatment you don't want. That includes treatment a physician recommends be started, and treatment that is already in use.

The reason this statement is important is that some people—including some physicians and nurses—who accept not starting life-sustaining treatment feel different about stopping ongoing treatment. They accept that death after not starting life-sustaining treatment occurs from natural causes, but they feel that death after stopping treatment is caused by human action.

Official ethics statements of major physician organizations, the judgment of the President's Commission for the Study of Ethical Problems in Medicine and Biomedical and Behavioral Research (in "Deciding to Forego Life-Sustaining Treatment"), and many court decisions hold that there is no ethical or legal difference between not starting unwanted treatment in the first place and stopping such treatment already in use. But many providers are not aware of these statements, or understand them intellectually but have a hard time applying them. And, some providers disagree with them.

3. *Treatment you do not want is not in your best interest.* The model documents encourage providers and others to see that the primary basis for determining your best interest should be *your* values about quality of life and medical treatment, not necessarily what is best in medical terms.

If possible, personalize the values statement by identifying any particular experiences or beliefs that influence the way you see the value of medical treatment. Sometimes physicians, nurses, and others resist accepting health-care planning statements that they see as being hypothetical. Personal statements can help to overcome such resistance by showing that your choices reflect personal experience.

Personalized statements are also important because they help your providers see that the documents you make really do reflect your values and choices. That kind of assurance can be particularly important when documents are entirely or partly printed, like the models in this book, because some physicians think patients don't understand what they read, or even sign forms without reading them. A personalizing statement helps answer such concerns.

Examples of personalizing statements might be knowledge that you have a serious health condition; personal experience with a serious illness or with life-sustaining treatment; or that you went through a terminal illness with a relative or close friend whose death was delayed by use of life supports. You can make your point in a few sentences. For example:

Two years ago I was diagnosed with non-Hodgkin's lymphoma, a cancer I know can be fatal. I underwent chemotherapy and am in remission, but I know the cancer can return. My experience and knowledge have caused me to consider very seriously how I would want to be treated if I were to become too sick to express my health-care decisions personally.

Or:

I have been diagnosed as HIV-positive. Friends of mine have died of AIDS. I know that much can be done, medically, to control HIV-related life-threatening conditions I might get, and I welcome that; but I also know that there are limits to what can be done. I want treatment that can help me continue my work. If I could not work, then I would not want life-sustaining treatment.

A statement can be as simple as this:

Last year I spent a lot of time visiting with my friend, Ed Smith, as he died in the hospital on a ventilator. I wouldn't want that to happen to me; I wouldn't want a machine used to prolong my dying.

You should mention any religious beliefs that are important to your treatment choices, because religious beliefs enjoy special legal protection. An example would be that as a devout person you do not fear death but accept it as an entry to eternal life. Religious statements can refer to a particular medical procedure (for example, blood transfusion, if your religious belief prohibits that; see discussion of "Transfusion of blood or blood products, to replace lost or diseased blood" later in this chapter). You should mention secular philosophical values that are important to you, as well, but you need to be aware that secular values do not enjoy the same special legal status as religious ones.

Power of attorney at 7 (Supplement at 3), "My choices concerning life-sustaining treatment." In this section you can tell your agents (and physicians and family) the circumstances under which you do *not* want life-sustaining treatment, and particular treatments you do not want.

Note that this section in the power of attorney differs from the corresponding supplement section in an important way. In the

power of attorney the section is intended as guidance for your agent, to help him make decisions for you. In the supplement the section in effect gives instructions for your physician to follow. The reason for the difference is that you know and choose your agent, but you and the physician who decides about life-sustaining treatment for you might be strangers. That said, you need to know that in practice (reinforced by the laws in Florida, Indiana, North Dakota, and Nevada), physicians treat directives more as permission than instruction. A physician decides what treatment she considers reasonable in particular circumstances. If a directive is consistent with her decision, she treats it as consent to act accordingly. If it conflicts, she may treat it as advisory and may not follow it. That course of action may be appropriate when a directive does not clearly apply, but some physicians suspend directives whenever they conflict with physician choice. Strong family support for your intentions can curb that. So can having a health-care power of attorney in addition to a directive or declaration.

Part A: "I have lived a long life and I am ready to accept death when it comes. For that reason, if I become unable to make my own health-care decisions, and I have or get a life-threatening condition, I want no life-sustaining treatment, even if the reason for such treatment might be completely reversible." This part is self-explanatory, but a word of warning is in order. While this choice might seem natural to people who make it, sometimes it is not to laypeople (especially younger relatives) and providers. Some people feel that this kind of choice must reflect depression, especially if the person who makes that choice is healthy for his age, and so should be overridden. Also, providers may worry that this is not a free choice but a result of coercion by self-interested relatives, or of pressure from a sense that older people have some kind of duty to make way for others. If you initial Part A, you should assure your family and your providers that you do so freely. Do that in person.

Part B: *"I consider my quality of life unacceptable, or only marginally acceptable, now. For that reason, if I become unable to make my own health-care decisions, and I have or get a life-threatening condition, I want no life-sustaining treatment, even if the reason for such treatment might be completely reversible."* A person may consider his quality of life to be very poor but choose to continue living. He might consider suicide unacceptable, or be physically unable to end his life. He may have other reasons to live. If you are inclined to initial Part B, it is extremely important that you explain in writing why you are doing so, and discuss your reasons with your physician and your agents, and preferably with your family. If you intend to initial that statement in the supplement (Appendix B), it is even more important that you explain your reasons, since your physician might have to rely on her judgment and your document, alone.

Discussion of this choice is essential for a few reasons:

- A physician needs to understand your reasons. A written explanation that seems clear to you might not be clear to him.
- A physician might be able to suggest medical treatment to help you that you're not aware of. That can happen even if another physician said nothing could be done. You don't have to accept available treatment, but if your agent, physician, and family know that you were aware of treatment options and refused them, they may be more likely to accept Part B as your choice.
- A physician might be able to suggest resources for increased emotional and social support that would help make your life better. In many communities there are well-established support groups for people who are living with certain diseases or impairments (and groups for their families as well).
- Initialing Part B might cause some people to be concerned about whether your choice reflects depression, especially suicidal depression. Many physicians and nurses think that a person who is depressed cannot make a valid decision to decline life-sustaining treatment—even when it is perfectly understandable that a person living with severe impairment would feel depressed. A physician or nurse who thinks Part B reflects depression or a suicidal outlook might question the validity of the entire document—not just adoption of this statement. That can create a risk of conflict with the agent, rejection of the agent's choice, and possibly rejection of the entire document.

If you initial Part B, you need to express your reasons explicitly and fully, to answer those concerns. Here is an example from the power of attorney of a person with very severe diabetes (of course, very often diabetes does not become so serious):

I have advanced diabetes, which severely impairs every aspect of my life. I feel sick all the time, and vomit daily, usually two or three times; my vision is severely diminished; I can walk only a few steps, with help; I feel weak all the time; and I experience insulin shock comas, because of blood sugar imbalances that result from my inability to keep food down, which require hospitalization and medical intervention to prevent death. I feel that my quality of life has worsened after recovery from earlier episodes of insulin shock. I am under the regular care of a physician, and have been for some time. Following his advice, I am taking an experimental medication to try to control the nausea and vomiting, but it does not work. My other impairments are not being treated, and are not treatable. Particularly, I cannot avoid insulin shock.

I value life, and I would like to live if I could have an acceptable quality of life. But, because of the losses from my disease, I judge my quality of life to be unacceptable. I understand that those losses will not diminish, but will stay the same or worsen, and that medical treatment cannot stop or reverse the course of my disease. Consequently, I direct as follows:

  a. If I experience any life-threatening condition—particularly including, but not limited to, what appears to be insulin shock—I direct that nothing be done to try to prevent or delay my death.

  b. I further direct that if I am not in a health-care facility when I next appear to go into insulin shock, 911 *not* be called. I direct this provision to my family, to any nurse attending me in my home, and to anyone else who knows of these instructions.

If you want to initial Part B and you do not have a physician who knows you well, consider consulting a lawyer knowledgeable about health-care planning issues about how best to make a record of your state of mind when making your document.

Part C, Qualities of life. Some people find the circumstances in Part C troubling to think about, while others don't. Even if they are difficult for you, you need to address them so that your agents, family members,

and physician can know what you would want.

If you initial any of Part C, you are saying, in effect, that you consider life in that condition to be worse than death. Therefore, if (1) because of illness or injury you become unable to make your own decisions; and (2) an unacceptable condition is present then, or occurs later; and (3) you then have or later get a life-threatening condition, you want to let nature take its course. You want to be kept comfortable, but you don't want medical treatment used to keep you alive.

Put a dash in any space you do not initial. A dash means that you *would* want life-sustaining treatment if the condition described to the right of the space were to occur. A dash is preferable to leaving a space blank, to avoid questions later about whether initials might have been inserted in a space after your document was signed.

For most people, the considerations that decisively affect their judgments about quality of life are awareness; ability to think and communicate; independence versus dependence; and management of severe pain. These are the focus of Part C. Statements 1 and 2, and potentially 3, express degrees of ability to be aware of and interact with other people. Statement 3 focuses on physical dependency. Statement 4 concerns pain and pain management.

The material that follows can help you clarify your wishes, talk with your physician about your options, and explain your choices to your providers, family, and agents.

Statement 1: "Unconsciousness (chronic coma or persistent vegetative state) from which ability to think and communicate probably will not be recovered, or, unconsciousness lasting [insert number] _____ *days, whichever occurs first."* Unconsciousness can result from many causes. Chronic coma and persistent vegetative state are terms for unconsciousness caused by severe brain injury (technically, they involve injury to different parts of the brain) from which recovery of awareness, and ability to think and communicate, practically never occur.

Statement 1 uses the term "unconsciousness," with "coma" and "persistent vegetative state" in parentheses, for three reasons. First, the focus is on quality of life, not medical diagnosis. Second, many physicians do not strictly differentiate between coma and persistent vegetative state, referring to all long-term unconsciousness as coma, chronic coma, vegetative coma, or other similar terms. Third, in several states the laws that authorize health-care planning documents use these terms.

The certainty with which permanence of unconsciousness can be determined in adults varies considerably depending on the cause, location, and extent of brain damage, and on how long it has persisted.

The period of time required to diagnose persistent vegetative state with certainty ranges from one to three months to as long as 12 months. Summarizing several research studies, the American Medical Association has said that "Cognitive recovery after six months is vanishingly rare in patients older than 50 years."

One cause of unconsciousness is brain injury from oxygen deprivation following cardiopulmonary arrest (heart and breathing failure). Again summarizing several studies, the American Medical Association has said that few people who are still unconscious a month after such an event ever recover awareness, and that "essentially none" recover after three months.

When persistent vegetative state has occurred, according to the American Academy of Neurology, consciousness never returns. The American Medical Association sees some slight chance of recovery: 1 in 1,000, or one-tenth of one percent. Even then, recovery usually is only to a minimal degree of consciousness, without ability to think or speak.

Usually people who recover from unconsciousness begin to recover within a few days of injury, and improve gradually day by day. Contrary to popular conception, instances in which people remain in deep coma for a long time, then suddenly and unexpectedly awake and start talking, are extremely rare.

When improvement occurs, its extent might not be known for 18 months after injury, and the extent of a person's adaptation to impairment might not be known for 24 months.

Physicians vary in their readiness to consider unconsciousness to be permanent. A major reason has to do with how much risk they are willing to accept that they might be wrong about whether any recovery will occur, and if so how much. Generally, physicians' risk tolerance involves medical factors, and information about what risk is acceptable to the patient. Would you want life-sustaining treatment to be continued until permanence appeared *virtually certain*? Or, would you want such treatment to be stopped if unconsciousness *probably* would be permanent, or if you *might* be left with major brain damage? Would you want life-sustaining treatment not to be used at all in the event of unconsciousness—even if unconsciousness might be reversible—because you feel you have lived long enough, or you feel that your present quality of life is unacceptable? Whatever your intentions, it is important that your physician—and your family and agents—understand them.

People without knowledge of neurology (some health-care professionals as well as laypeople) may think that comatose people are not completely unconscious because of certain behaviors. People in deep coma appear to be continuously asleep, but sometimes stir or open their eyes, and may respond to noxious stimuli. People who are in a persistent vegetative state have sleep-wake cycles. Their eyes tear. Sometimes they turn their eyes toward sounds or movement, make sounds (when they are touched or moved, and at other times), make facial expressions (which can include what look like brief smiles), blink, and move their limbs. People who see that may feel that such actions must indicate awareness. They may also think that a person who has entered a persistent vegetative state from coma has improved, because of the change from a sleep-like state to making occasional movements and sounds. People involved in decision making need to know that these behaviors in a person in chronic coma are not intentional; they are reflexes, like leg or foot movement when a physician hits a knee tendon or Achilles tendon with a rubber hammer during a physical examination.

Based on evidence from clinical observation, autopsy, and brain function testing, the American Academy of Neurology and the American Medical Association have concluded that people who are in a persistent vegetative state have no awareness of any kind, including pain. There is no evidence to the contrary, although some physicians consider the evidence inconclusive because they believe it does not absolutely rule out possibility of awareness.

Persistent vegetative state and chronic coma are conditions that have been *created* by modern medicine, because without life-sustaining treatment unconscious people soon die. Virtually all people in these conditions get artificial nutrition and hydration. Many in coma, and some in persistent vegetative state, need machines to breathe for them. Most need antibiotics, because they develop infections (especially pneumonia and urinary tract infections) that can become life-threatening. Even with antibiotics most people in a persistent vegetative state or coma eventually die from some infection; this happens because reflexes that in healthy people clear the throat and lungs are absent, which increases the risk of respiratory infection. Other life-sustaining medications besides antibiotics are often needed to control heart function, blood pressure, blood sugar, and convulsions.

People with long-term unconsciousness almost always are in nursing homes, but at some point most are transferred to hospitals because of acute problems that nursing homes cannot manage. About 60 percent of unconscious nursing home residents are sent to hospitals at some point, and about 30 percent are moved multiple times.

Statement 1 includes the words "from which ability to think and communicate probably will not be recovered" to limit the length of time that life-sustaining treatment would be used if you were to become unconscious. Thinking and communication imply full, or nearly full, recovery. Often that possibility can be ruled out long before the chance of recovery to some lower level of consciousness.

Statement 1 lets you specify the number of days of unconsciousness after which you would want life-sustaining treatment to be stopped even if your physician is not yet ready to say that you will never regain awareness. Many people would want life-sustaining treatment to be continued until their physician decides their condition is permanent. If that is what you want, then put a dash in the space to the left of "days" at C 1. Other people prefer to state a maximum number of days for use of such treatment, because they fear being sustained indefinitely if their physician won't predict permanence, or because they want to spare their family lengthy uncertainty or expense. If you want life-sustaining treatment to stop after a certain time, even if your medical situation remains uncertain, put a number in the appropriate space.

If you insert a time limit, you need to discuss it with your physician, because your limit might not make medical sense. That does not make it invalid; you might have good personal reasons for wanting life-sustaining treatment to stop after a certain time. But, a physician might not accept your time limit without understanding your reasons. Even then he might not accept it; if that happens and you have an agent, the agent can decide whether to allow life-sustaining treatment to continue or to change physicians. If you do not have an agent, but have only a directive or declaration, then you may have to depend on your physician to accept your time limit.

If you initial the space to the left of the "Unconsciousness" option and insert a number in the space before "days," you are telling your agent and physician that if you become unconscious then you do not want life-sustaining treatment beyond that number of days. Looking at it another way, you are telling your agent that she can allow life-sustaining treatment for that long to see if

consciousness returns. As with other decisions in Section 7, the model power of attorney gives an agent guidance, not absolute instructions. So, unless you change the model document to direct that life-sustaining treatment stop after a certain period of time, your agent will decide whether to continue treatment longer than the period you indicate if she believes there is a good enough reason to do so.

Note that in Ohio, if you intend a living will to be implemented in the event of permanent unconsciousness your document must use the term "permanently unconscious state" and define it in a certain way. To comply with the law, in the supplement at Statement 1 before the word "Unconsciousness" insert the words "Permanently unconscious state"; then attach the "Statement Regarding 'Terminal Condition' and 'Permanently Unconscious State'" from Appendix D, under Ohio. (For powers of attorney, attach the Ohio notice from Appendix D.)

Statement 2: "Brain damage that probably is not reversible, and causes apparently complete, or nearly complete, loss of ability to think or communicate." This statement describes impairment short of unconsciousness, that can result from serious illness or injury.

Determining when such a condition is present requires subjective judgments by both your physician and your agent. How *much* loss is complete, or nearly complete? How do they know, from what they see, what loss has actually occurred? How certain do they have to be that apparent losses are permanent? This choice is included because it is one that many people want to make. But, for it to work as you intend you may need to explain just what you mean to your physicians, family, and agents.

Statement 3: "Total dependence on others for care, because of deterioration that probably is not reversible." Total dependence for care can develop suddenly (for example, from a major stroke), or over time (for example, from a degenerative neurological disease). For some people life with complete physical dependence is not worth living. Other people feel different, especially if they can still communicate.

If you initial Statement 3, be sure to tell all concerned how sure you would want them to be that total dependence is permanent before deciding not to start, or to stop, life-sustaining treatment. Do you have in mind something like 51 percent, 99 percent, or something in between?

Statement 4: "Pain control that is inadequate, either because pain cannot be eliminated, or because the amount of medicine needed to eliminate pain causes so much sedation that ability to communicate verbally is lost." Usually pain can be controlled (by pain medication, and/or by treating whatever is causing the pain), but sometimes it cannot be eliminated. Also, medication for severe pain can cause sedation, sometimes to the point of unconsciousness or near-unconsciousness. Statement 4 expresses the choice that for someone who can no longer speak personally, being free from pain is more important than perhaps living longer with pain or in a heavily sedated state.

When sedation is a problem, sometimes awareness can be restored by reducing pain medication. Then the patient can decide personally whether to start or continue life-sustaining treatment instead of an agent having to decide. At other times, though, that cannot be done because the resulting pain would prevent decision making.

Note that this option does not require that pain be permanent. Sometimes disabling pain is permanent, but often it is not. When it is not, duration can vary widely, from minutes to months. The main situation for which this option is intended is severe pain caused by advanced cancer, but it can apply in other situations. Whether to stop or not to start life-sustaining treatment because of pain issues requires an agent to exercise judgment.

Statement 5: Other circumstances in which you do not want life-sustaining treatment. If there are circumstances in which you do not want such treatment other than those described in C 1 through 4, describe them here.

The question of "terminal condition." Most people think, at first, that whether they would want life-sustaining treatment depends on whether they are dying from a terminal condition. Why, then, isn't terminal condition mentioned in the model documents as a reason to limit use of life-sustaining treatment?

There are three reasons. First, many people tend to think that whether a condition is or is not terminal is a fact that physicians can determine with certainty at any time, but often this is not the case. Second, people have different ideas about how soon death is expected to occur for a condition to be considered terminal. Some fatal conditions can exist for years before death occurs. Third, presence of a fatal condition does not necessarily mean that quality of life is poor. For both providers and laypeople, whether a condition is considered terminal often involves nonmedical value judgments about what makes life worth living. Statements that medical treatment "prolongs life" or "prolongs dying" can reflect such value judgments.

Requiring that health-care planning documents be used only if a terminal condition has been diagnosed can make physicians feel obligated to use life-sustaining treatments until every uncertainty has disappeared. Often that means life supports are used until the patient dies.

To many laypeople the significance of concluding that a condition is terminal is that life-sustaining treatment stop. Even then, however, physicians may still offer such treatment. Life-sustaining treatment might be offered to cure some other, more immediate life-threatening condition. For example, a physician might recommend antibiotic treatment for a person with potentially fatal pneumonia who also has incurable cancer. Or treatment might be offered to relieve a symptom, such as pain from a cancerous tumor, but have the additional effect of lengthening life.

Having heard all that, if you want your agent to make certain decisions only if you have a terminal condition, by all means say so; you are making *your* document. Just be sure to tell your agents, physicians, and family what "terminal" means to you.

Note that in Ohio, if you intend a living will to be implemented because of a "terminal condition" you must use that term and define it in a certain way. To comply with the law, in the supplement write your intention in the space provided in Section 2, then attach to your document the "Statement Regarding 'Terminal Condition' and 'Permanently Unconscious State'" from Appendix D, under Ohio. (For powers of attorney, attach the Ohio notice from Appendix D.)

Section 7 D, "Particular life-sustaining treatments." Here you should identify particular life-sustaining treatments that you authorize your agent to reject.

It is important for you to understand that in the power of attorney this part does not require your agent to reject certain treatments; it authorizes him to do so when he believes that is what you would want.

In the supplement this section *is* framed as instructions. In practice, though, it will operate much like a power of attorney; if a physician feels an instruction is wrong in current circumstances she will probably suspend it.

It is also important for you to let your providers know that this is not a strict treatment rejection list. Many physicians believe that laypeople are not competent to reject particular life-sustaining treatments. Tell your physician your document includes a treatment list because:

- You are concerned that if decisions need to be made for you the physician in charge of your case at the time might not know you, and might want to see express authorization.
- You want to enable your agent to make difficult choices, and to make them as you intend. Expressly authorizing rejection of particular treatments can help him do so.
- You want to help members of your family accept decisions your agent makes.
- In some states the law requires such strict proof of intention to reject life-sustaining treatment (especially artificial nutrition and hydration) that anything less than naming unwanted treatments might be inadequate. You want to be sure to meet the most stringent legal standard that can be applied to your agent's decisions.

As you consider your treatment choices, keep in mind that your agent will have authority to make decisions if you are unable to do so.

In the Durable Power of Attorney for Health-Care Decisions you initial each treatment in Section 7 D (3 D in the supplement) unless you definitely want it. If you do not initial a treatment that your agent later wants to reject on your behalf, someone might oppose his decision in the belief that since you did not initial the particular treatment you did not intend your agent to have authority to reject it. Similarly, you should initial each treatment in the supplement that you want your physician to withhold.

Confusion can arise if you initial 7 A, B, or C but don't initial every treatment in Section 7 D. Section 7 says that for the reason you initialed, you would not want any life-sustaining treatment. Putting a dash in any part of Section 7 D contradicts that by saying you might want that particular treatment. It is more important that your document reflect your intentions than that it be perfectly logically consistent, but people need to be fairly certain of what your intentions are. So, if you put a dash next to any treatment in 7 D (3 D in the supplement)—or if you change the model to say that you definitely want a certain life-sustaining treatment—you should attach a written explanation to your document. As important as this is for a power of attorney, it can be crucial for a directive or declaration, which does not name an agent; there might not be a person available who knows what you meant, or that person's explanation might not be reliable in the eyes of your physician, the facility attorney, or a judge. So, be sure to explain what you intend as clearly as possible.

As you read through the treatment list you might feel unsure about whether to initial a particular choice. You might want a treatment for a limited period, to try to restore health or at least reverse some disease process, but not want it to continue indefinitely. Or, you might be unsure whether or not you would want a treatment at all. If so, initial the treatment, then initial the first option at "Temporary use of life-sustaining treatment," Section 7 E of the power of attorney and Section 3 E of the supplement. If you are sure that you would not want even trial use of life-sustaining treatment, you can say that by initialing the second option at 7 E and 3 E.

The model documents are structured so your treatment choices apply uniformly to all qualities of life that you decide are unacceptable. This approach suits many people, but not everyone. Some people want certain treatments in some circumstances but not others. If this is true for you, then you should explain that in your documents. Be sure to discuss such wishes with your physician before your documents are put in final form.

> **Note:** The purpose of the following discussion about particular treatments is to give you information for talking with your physician about health-care planning. You should not rely on this information alone. General, written information cannot take the place of face-to-face discussion with a physician, especially one who knows your health situation and whom you trust. Discussion can help you be sure about what you want, and can help your providers understand your intentions.

"Nutrition and hydration, other than ordinary food and water by mouth if I cannot eat and drink, at all or enough to sustain me." If you initial the space to the left of this statement, you are telling your agent that if you initialed Section 7 A or B, or any part of 7 C, and you ever have a life-threatening condition, then you do *not* want artificial nutrition and hydration.

Severe injury or disease can make people lose the ability or desire to eat and drink, to get the necessary nutrition from food, or to take in as much nutrition orally as the body needs. When that happens, life often can be sustained by artificial nutrition and hydration. Use of artificial nutrition and hydration can be temporary or permanent, depending on the medical circumstances.

"Artificial" refers to both the substances given and the way in which they are delivered. The substances are chemical nutrients mixed in a liquid. They are delivered either by an intravenous line (usually into a vein in the chest), or by a nasogastric tube (a tube down the nose into the stomach), or by a surgically implanted tube (through the abdomen into the stomach or an intestine).

When artificial nutrition and hydration are needed but not provided, death results either from heart failure brought on by dehydration (people can live much longer without nutrition than hydration), or from the condition that caused the loss of ability or desire to eat and drink in the first place. Death from dehydration occurs within about three days to two weeks.

Many people assume that withholding or withdrawing artificial nutrition and hydration is uncomfortable, and that providing them gives comfort. This is sometimes true. A person who is generally healthy and alert but cannot eat or drink for some days before and after stomach surgery, for example, would feel hungry and thirsty without artificial nutrition and hydration, and would need them to return to health. Even near the end of life, artificial hydration can sometimes increase alertness, contribute to a sense of well-being, and decrease nausea that might be present (although nausea often can be lessened by medication). But at other times, a person may not experience artificial nutrition and hydration as beneficial. Sometimes these measures can even cause suffering, when withholding or withdrawing them would relieve suffering.

Every experienced family physician has seen people who are physically able to eat and drink choose to stop as they near death, then die without showing any sign of hunger or thirst. Dehydration and undernutrition cause the body to make natural pain-relieving substances. (This can reduce the need for pain medicines.) When body fluids decrease, which often occurs as death nears, not replenishing them can reduce nausea related to underlying disease.

In contrast, sometimes artificial nutrition and hydration cause discomfort. The way artificial nutrition and hydration are given, particularly by nasogastric tube, can cause significant discomfort, and frequently results in aspiration pneumonia (breathing fluid into the lungs). Patients sometimes pull out nasogastric tubes; then they may be physically restrained or heavily sedated to prevent repeated removal. Restraints can cause further discomfort and suffering.

Artificial nutrition can cause nausea, diarrhea and other problems (which can be avoided by adjusting the nutrition, but must be tolerated in the meantime). Artificial hydration increases secretions that people who are experiencing respiratory depression (common near the end of life) cannot clear themselves, making breathing difficult. These secretions can be suctioned, but the suctioning itself can be uncomfortable or painful, and sometimes cannot be done as often as needed. Hydration also can aggravate edema or pressure from some tumors.

Artificial nutrition and hydration also sometimes keep a person alert enough to be aware of approaching death. Some people value or accept that, while for others that awareness can be deeply distressing.

Some people who have severe physical impairments that prevent eating come to feel that continued life offers nothing meaningful to them, and that artificial nutrition and hydration sustain them only to suffer. They sometimes choose to stop, either personally when they are conscious, or through health-care planning documents after consciousness has been lost.

Finally, for people in a persistent vegetative state or chronic coma there is no reason to believe that artificial nutrition and hydration provide any benefit.

Some people—including physicians and nurses—who accept withholding and withdrawing other life-sustaining treatments feel different about artificial nutrition and hydration. Many physicians and nurses believe that artificial nutrition and hydration should always be provided. Some will agree not to start them, but refuse to stop them later. Likewise, many nursing homes, and some hospitals, have policies that prohibit withholding and/or withdrawal. Disputes about this can become highly emotional; whether or not a person will benefit from getting artificial nutrition and hydration, many people (health-care providers and laypeople alike) feel that they must give them.

Providers' openness to rejection of artificial nutrition and hydration also can be influenced by legal considerations. Some laws that authorize health-care planning documents exclude artificial nutrition and hydration from treatments that can be withheld or withdrawn in reliance on such documents, and providers may be unaware that patients have other, broader rights to refuse unwanted treatment, including these measures. Also, several living will and health-care power of attorney laws say that patient comfort measures must always be provided. Whether artificial nutrition and hydration contribute to comfort can be unclear, so a provider may hesitate to withhold or withdraw them from fear of legal repercussions despite her patient's wishes. Also, some physicians and nurses claim that artificial nutrition and hydration are always needed for comfort. Finally, in some states laws intended to guard against abuse of the elderly and laws that regulate nursing homes can discourage withholding or withdrawing artificial nutrition and hydration even from patients who have said they do not want them.

If at all possible, you should determine a physician's attitude and a facility's policy regarding artificial nutrition and hydration before beginning a relationship with them. Talk with your physician. Ask whether a facility has a written policy allowing withholding and withdrawing of life-sustaining treatment generally, and artificial nutrition and hydration specifically. If so, get a copy. If a facility does not have a written policy that accepts your wishes, you should investigate other options.

"All cardiopulmonary resuscitation measures, to try to restart my heart and

breathing if those stop." If you initial the space to the left of this statement, you are telling your agent and providers that if you are already in a condition that you said in Section 7 C is unacceptable to you, and you initialed 7 A or 7 B, and your heart or breathing stops, you do *not* want cardiopulmonary resuscitation.

Usually if either breathing or circulation stops the other stops soon after. If both are stopped for too long the brain dies, and the person is considered dead. Sometimes circulation and/or breathing that have stopped can be restarted. First air is breathed into the affected person's lungs and the chest is rhythmically compressed and released. The principle is that a heart that is basically sound will start beating effectively if it gets oxygenated blood. Breathing moves oxygen into the bloodstream and chest compression circulates the oxygenated blood to the heart and brain. (If air cannot get to the lungs a tube may be put down the throat so air can get through. This is called intubation.) If breathing and compression don't work, certain medications are injected. If they don't work, a controlled electric shock (called defibrillation) is administered. If heartbeat and breathing can be restarted further life support is often needed, especially mechanical ventilation (breathing by machine) and medications. A common name for resuscitation procedures is "CPR," for "cardiopulmonary resuscitation."

Resuscitation was originally used to prevent sudden, unexpected death from heart or breathing stoppage, particularly related to anesthesia during surgery. It was intended for people who were thought to be healthy but whose circulation or breathing had stopped because of surgical events. Over time, however, a presumption developed that it should be used whenever circulation or breathing stops, no matter what the person's health. Now, to many physicians, almost everyone is a candidate for resuscitation.

Why would anyone *not* want resuscitation? Some people feel they have lived a long and good life, and are ready to accept death when it comes. Some other people feel their quality of life is so poor that they do not want to be "saved" to continue in that condition, or worse. These issues aside, resuscitation simply does not work very often or very well, especially on people who are very sick when their heart or breathing fails.

Resuscitation outcomes are especially poor when heart failure results from irreversible illness or severe deterioration of one or more organ systems. Research findings show that when hospitalized patients whose hearts stop get resuscitation, about one-third (33 percent to 39 percent) survive the effort. In other words, about two-thirds of the time hearts cannot be restarted. (In nursing homes, outcomes probably are worse than in hospitals, because advanced technology and specialized personnel are less available, and because resuscitation often is not started as quickly.) Of the third who are resuscitated, only a third of those (in other words, 11 percent to 17 percent of the total on whom resuscitation is tried) survive to discharge from the hospital (including discharge to a nursing home). The chance of surviving to discharge depends very much on particular health factors. Other studies have found that of hospitalized patients with metastatic cancer, pneumonia, or acute stroke with neurologic deficit on whom resuscitation is tried, none survived to discharge. Among patients with renal (kidney) failure 2 percent survived to discharge. For sepsis (severe bacterial infection of the blood or tissues), the discharge rate was less than 1 percent. (Note that while serious illness impairs the chance of restoring heart function, there is no clear evidence that advancing age does.)

Another consideration, besides whether heart function can be restored, is the quality of life of people who survive resuscitation but then do not live to be discharged from the hospital. They almost always spend their remaining time in an intensive care unit, often with invasive treatments and monitoring. These often include mechanical ventilation, which prevents speech. The usual intensive care unit environment can make communication and privacy difficult.

Resuscitation efforts can directly worsen quality of life. Unless normal heartbeat and breathing are restored quickly, permanent brain damage can occur. Such damage can affect ability to think, and/or to control various bodily functions, including breathing, speech, and use of limbs. The extent of damage depends on how long the brain is deprived of oxygen, the reason heartbeat and/or breathing stopped, and sometimes other circumstances. Brain damage can begin in four minutes; irreversible, total unconsciousness can occur in six minutes. Often health-care providers do not know how long heart function and breathing have been stopped when resuscitation is started. Also, health-care providers often continue resuscitation much longer than four to six minutes, until heart function is restored or death is declared. Of everyone on whom CPR is attempted, about 2 percent to 2.7 percent end up in a persistent vegetative state—a probability that for many patients is as great, or greater than, the probability that their hearts can be restarted at all. If brain damage occurs withdrawal of life support may not be an option; it is possible for a person to be severely brain damaged but not need life support. People who are left with significant impairment almost always go to nursing homes.

Besides brain damage, resuscitation efforts can cause damage to internal organs, the aspiration of stomach contents into the lungs (which can result in permanent dependence on a breathing machine), and fractured ribs.

Witnessing resuscitation efforts and a poor aftermath can be terribly hard for a patient's family. That can be true for providers, too, especially when they know the chance of recovery is very poor.

For one or more of these reasons, many people choose not to undergo resuscitation.

Refusing resuscitation requires special preparation, because it is an emergency procedure. Decisions about whether to use other life-sustaining treatments often can be discussed for some time, but resuscitation has to be begun right away. For that reason virtually all health-care facilities have special procedures for starting it immediately, without requesting consent from anyone. Even if someone present when heartbeat or breathing stops and says not to attempt resuscitation, she will be ignored unless the person whose responsibility it is to start the procedure knows that she really has the authority to refuse it; he cannot take the time to find out whether she does or not. The law supports that practice; when a life-threatening emergency occurs the law presumes consent would be given, so that potentially life-saving treatment can begin without delay. In some states (Georgia, Indiana, Iowa, Mississippi, New Jersey, North Dakota, Ohio, Tennessee, West Virginia, and Wyoming), the laws direct or imply that health-care planning documents routinely be suspended during emergencies.

Resuscitation will only be withheld if an attending physician has made a written order to that effect. The order usually is called a "no-code order," "DNR order" (for "do not resuscitate"), or "DNAR order" (for "do not attempt resuscitation").

If you do not want resuscitation, you should request a DNAR order from your physician yourself, if you are able to make your own decisions, or tell your agent to request such an order if you lose decision-making capacity and you experience a quality of life in which you would not want your life to be sustained. Don't wait for your physician to raise the subject; that might never happen.

Do not assume that a DNAR order will be entered automatically even in the event of grave illness. On the other hand, some physicians may enter a DNAR order without discussion or disclosure if they believe that CPR would be "futile." That view is controversial (because futility judgments are supposed to be objective, but in fact often involve physicians' value judgments about what effort is worth making). If your physician won't discuss resuscitation, or expresses values that don't fit with yours, then you should change physicians.

Only a physician—never a nurse—can enter a DNAR order. But you (or if you are incapacitated, your agent) should be sure to discuss your wishes with your regular nurses, too. If a nurse doesn't accept that a patient should not be resuscitated, she might resist or avoid a DNAR order. Just as with physicians, talking with nurses about your wishes can help bring about understanding and acceptance of your choices.

Be aware that a DNAR order, once entered, might not continue throughout a hospitalization; an order may be revoked if the attending physician believes the patient's condition has improved. For that reason, if the patient's condition fluctuates during a hospitalization or nursing home stay, resuscitation status needs to be discussed from time to time.

DNAR orders almost never carry over from one hospitalization to a later hospitalization, and usually do not transfer from one facility to another.

If you are not in a health-care facility but are anticipating entering one (for example, a nursing home or hospice, or a hospital for planned surgery), request that their DNAR policy be explained to you, and ask to see their written policy. Since 1988, every accredited hospital has been required to have a written policy regarding use of resuscitation. Many nursing homes have such policies as well.

Note: A DNAR order applies only to resuscitation, but some physicians and nurses treat rejection of resuscitation as rejection of other life-sustaining measures. If you do not want resuscitation but do want other life-sustaining treatment, make sure your providers understand that. Also, because resuscitation involves multiple procedures, physicians can have different ideas about just what a DNAR order covers. You should reach an understanding with your physician about this.

Once a DNAR order is entered, a health-care facility should have a procedure in place for assuring that key people know about it. Procedures don't always work, though. Communication can break down. Realistically, you can't do much about procedural risks short of your agent or a family member being present more or less constantly and asking every physician and nurse whether she knows a no-code order has been entered. If a facility's written DNAR policy includes procedures for follow-through, an order may be more likely to be communicated.

Some surgeons and anesthesiologists, and some hospital policies, routinely suspend DNAR orders during surgery. One major reason is that normal anesthesiology practices (breathing for the patient, and regulating heart function) can be difficult to distinguish from resuscitation, so a DNAR order can be difficult to follow. Another reason is that surgery and anesthesia increase the risk of heart and breathing failure, and failures during surgery often are reversible. Still, there can be a compelling reason to continue a DNAR order during surgery: when the person undergoing surgery judges his health condition to be so poor, even considering whatever benefit surgery might provide, that if arrest were to occur he would not want to be resuscitated. An example is arrest during surgery to remove a painful, cancerous tumor that will recur, and ultimately will be fatal. In that circumstance some people want to be resuscitated while others do not.

If you want surgery but do not want resuscitation, you need to talk with your surgeon and anesthesiologist near the time of the operation. (If you cannot speak for yourself, then your agent, if you have one, should do so for you. Rarely will a living will be enough to keep a DNAR order in effect during surgery.) Talking with your family physician or a nurse is not good enough. When an operation is not an emergency, the surgeon should meet with you (or your agent, if you are incapacitated) in ad-

vance to discuss the procedure and request consent. That is a good time to talk with him, and to ask that he have the anesthesiologist see you.

If you know that you might undergo resuscitation during surgery—either because you agree to it, or because your physicians are not willing to accept a DNAR order—be sure to discuss how long such measures might be continued after surgery. Sometimes when breathing and heart function stop during surgery and heartbeat is restored, mechanical ventilation must be used because breathing ability remains impaired. (In that situation, ventilation is considered part of the resuscitation effort.) The cause can be either continuing effects of surgery, or a disease process that was present before the surgery. In most cases that can be determined within 24 to 48 hours. Whatever the cause of inability to breathe, would you want mechanical ventilation to be continued after surgery at all, and if so for how long? Many physicians do not cover this in a general discussion of surgery and anesthesia, even though the problem is very real. If you are concerned about being on a ventilator after surgery, be sure to discuss that with your physicians.

Also be sure that any understanding about use of resuscitation measures after surgery is written down in your chart, because after surgery your surgeon and anesthesiologist may no longer be in charge of your care.

If you do not want resuscitation and you live in an area that has a 911 emergency response system, you should consider whether you would want 911 to be called. In most places, if 911 is called resuscitation will be done unless it is obviously hopeless, even if the emergency medical technicians are told that the person whose heart has stopped does not want it. The main reason is the same as in a hospital: there isn't time to determine the patient's intention or the authority of the person who claims to represent the patient's wishes.

Note: In some places emergency providers can withhold resuscitation, while still providing other emergency medical care (such as medications to relieve anxiety, pain, and breathing difficulty), if necessary arrangements have been made in advance. That is allowed by law in Arizona, Colorado, Florida, Montana, New York, Pennsylvania, and Virginia, by policy in Maine, Maryland, Massachusetts, New Jersey, Wyoming, and the District of Columbia, and some localities in California and elsewhere. The list probably will grow. Various restrictions apply. If you would want emergency medical treatment, but not resuscitation, check with your local emergency medical services provider to find out what is possible in your area, then discuss the options with your physician.

If you do not want 911 to be called, you should tell anyone whom you would expect to be in the position of calling (people who regularly visit you, neighbors, etc.). You should tell those same people not to try to resuscitate you themselves.

"Mechanical ventilation (breathing by machine), if I am unlikely to recover the ability to breathe in my own without it." If you initial the space to the left of this statement, you are telling your agent that if you initialed Section 7 A or B, or any part of 7 C, and you ever have a life-threatening condition, you do *not* want mechanical ventilation.

Mechanical ventilation involves putting a tube into the lung area, then pumping oxygen through the tube. Usually the tube is fed through the nose or mouth and then down the trachea or windpipe. When ventilation is expected to be long-term, the tube is placed through a hole made in the trachea (this is called a tracheostomy). Aside from sustaining life, mechanical ventilation can relieve discomfort caused by breathing insufficiency.

Like resuscitation, mechanical ventilation was originally used only for patients who were expected to regain ability to breathe on their own, but over time its use has expanded to include everyone who cannot breathe sufficiently without it. Often it is needed only temporarily. But when normal breathing cannot be restored, a person either remains on mechanical ventilation until death occurs (which in some cases can be years), or ventilation is withdrawn and the person dies. When mechanical ventilation is withdrawn, death usually occurs in a few minutes to 24 hours, depending on the person's health, but can take considerably longer. During that time, medications can be given to prevent anxiety or physical discomfort related to the withdrawal.

"Surgeries that would prolong my life." If you initial the space to the left of this statement, you are telling your agent and providers that if you initialed Section 7 A or B, or any part of 7 C, and you ever have a life-threatening condition, then you do *not* want your life prolonged by surgery.

Physicians often recommend surgery that serves the valid medical goal of eliminating an immediate threat to life, but that might or might not restore an acceptable quality of life. A person who is severely demented and gets an operable cancer, for example, will still be severely demented after the tumor is removed. Whether life-sustaining surgery is a good thing depends on how you see the length and quality of life the surgery will permit. For example, surgery to remove a cancerous bowel tumor after the cancer has spread to other sites buys time; but it can cause loss of function, which some people tolerate well but others do not. And, because the cancer will continue to grow, the person may have to decide in the future whether to remove other organs, with more loss of function. Knowing that, some people would choose surgery; others would not.

Sometimes surgery that is intended to improve quality of remaining life also prolongs life. A physician might offer surgery as a way to improve quality of life, for example, by eliminating a source of pain. But pain relief may be achievable by medication without surgery.

As with other treatment decisions an agent might need to make, decisions about surgery can require that he find his way through a thicket of information and conflicting goals. Keeping an eye on your quality of life choices can help him find his way.

"Dialysis or filtration, to clean life-threatening substances from my blood." If you initial the space to the left of this statement, you are telling your agent that if you initialed Section 7 A or B, or any part of 7 C, and you ever have a life-threatening condition, you do *not* want dialysis or filtration to be started, or if already in use, you want it stopped.

In all healthy people blood circulates through the kidneys, which filter out potentially dangerous substances. When kidneys fail, blood cleaning can be done mechanically. Usually the procedure involves cir-culating the blood from a vessel (commonly in the arm) through a small tube into a cleaning machine and then back into the vessel. Dialysis and filtration work differently, technically, but serve the same purpose and are similar in terms of patient experience. The process typically is done about three times a week for four to eight hours each time, although frequency and duration can vary. Sometimes blood cleaning is needed only temporarily, to allow kidneys to heal from disease or injury. Usually the need is permanent, unless a kidney is successfully transplanted. (A person needs only one healthy kidney to live normally.) If both kidneys suddenly fail and dialysis is not started, or if dialysis is stopped, death results, usually within hours to three days. Death from sudden kidney failure or from stopping dialysis is painless. When the kidneys fail gradually, death can take up to two weeks. Gradual kidney failure causes seriously distressing symptoms, which require heavy medication to control.

Long-term dialysis can be stressful for patients and their families. Dialysis can cause significant physical problems, and related psychological stress. When dialysis is done at home, patients and families sometimes feel burdened and isolated. Also at home, the very presence of the machinery, and its use, can be stressful. How well people cope with such problems varies. Anyone considering starting long-term dialysis should discuss potential difficulties with their provider.

You need to be aware that if you personally accept dialysis or filtration, and later become unable to speak for yourself, your agent or family can have difficulty stopping it. They might feel that since you consented to it they should not withdraw consent. A provider might be unwilling to accept their withdrawal for the same reason. To head off such problems, you need to make clear to your family, agents, and providers that if you accept dialysis you do so because of the quality of life it permits, and that if your quality of life were to become unacceptable then the reason for your consent would no longer apply.

"Transfusion of blood or blood products, to replace lost or diseased blood." If you initial the space to the left of this statement, you are telling your agent that if you initialed Section 7 A or B, or any part of 7 C, and you ever have a life-threatening condition, you do *not* want transfusion of blood or blood products.

Transfusion of blood or blood products replaces blood that has been lost by injury, or that is unable to perform its function because of disease or genetic defect. Blood is transfused through a needle into a vein. Transfusions may be administered only once, or may have to be repeated over time, depending on the circumstances.

Transfusion can sometimes return a person to full health. An example would be transfusion to replace blood loss due to injuries sustained in an automobile collision. In other circumstances transfusion may extend life but not eliminate an underlying life-threatening condition (although some other treatment given at the same time might be able to do that). An example would be transfusions to replace red blood cells in someone who has lymphoma (a kind of cancer) and is receiving chemotherapy; transfusion can provide needed blood, while chemotherapy is given in an attempt to cure the cancer. Sometimes transfusions are used to treat pain (for example, from sickle cell ane-

mia). Finally, sometimes transfusions are given solely to extend life during progression of a fatal disease.

Transfusion poses various risks, related to the transfused blood itself and to the transfusion process. Blood-related risks include allergic and other reactions, and transmission of viral and bacterial diseases, which can be significant and unavoidable. Process risks include infection and physical injuries, which are avoidable if careful techniques are used by medical personnel.

If you reject blood transfusion on religious grounds, express that in the space at the end of the values statement (Section 6 of the power of attorney; Section 2 of the supplement). If, within your beliefs, certain *methods* of blood transfer, or *kinds* of blood or blood substitute products, are acceptable to you while others are not, be sure to explain that. If you want life-sustaining treatments *other* than blood transfusion to be withheld or withdrawn only if your quality of life becomes unacceptable, but you refuse blood transfusions no matter what your quality of life or medical condition, say that. Also be sure to initial the space by "Transfusion of blood or blood products, to replace lost or diseased blood" in Section 7 D of the power of attorney and Section 3 D of the supplement.

"Medications, when the purpose is to cure or control life-threatening conditions rather than control pain (for example: antibiotics, chemotherapy, insulin)." If you initial the space to the left of this statement, you are telling your agent that if you initialed Section 7 A or B, or any part of 7 C, and you ever have a life-threatening condition, you want life-sustaining medication *not* to be started, or if already in use to be stopped.

Medications commonly are life-sustaining in three circumstances: (1) when they replace some substance the body needs, such as insulin, hormones, or steroids, allowing essentially full quality of life; (2) when they are intended to cure, but whether cure will occur is uncertain; and (3) when they have no potential to cure, but are used only to prolong life.

In all three circumstances use of medication can conflict with concerns about quality of life. Replacement therapy can keep a person alive who is suffering from some unrelated condition. Curative medication can directly cause suffering, in hope of producing an uncertain cure. For example, some kinds of chemotherapy can make people terribly sick, or even cause death. Medicine in the third category can neither cure nor relieve suffering, but only buy time.

Conditions that are treated by life-sustaining medications do not always cause discomfort, so withholding or withdrawing such medications need not involve discomfort, either. When discomfort is an issue, often symptoms can be controlled by other medications that are not life-sustaining.

"Anything else that sustains, restores, or replaces a vital body function." The purpose of this option is to head off objections that once you start to specify treatments you don't want, no treatment can be withheld or withdrawn unless it is on your list. You cannot list every treatment that could be used to sustain life. Initialing this option reinforces your agent's authority to make decisions for you.

Section 7 E, "Temporary use of life-sustaining treatment." Some people simply do not want life-sustaining treatment at all. Other people want such treatment if it offers a reasonably good chance of improving their health, but are afraid that once such treatment starts it will be continued indefinitely.

This part lets you tell your agent and physician if you would want life-sustaining treatment on a trial basis, to see if it would be helpful. Again, be sure to discuss this with your physician.

This part also allows you to set a flexible time limit. A time limit serves the aim of avoiding your being maintained on life supports in circumstances you consider unacceptable, and gives emotional permission to all who are concerned about you to stop life support efforts if improvement does not occur within the time frame you indicate. The time limit is flexible because you could be improving when your limit is reached, but not have improved sufficiently to stop support. If you might want trial use of life-sustaining treatment, and you trust your agent enough to authorize that, you should trust her to bend a time limit, too. An approximate duration can help her decide how long is long enough. Talking to her about this provision can help her even more.

The situation is more difficult with a directive or declaration, because decisions might be made for you by a stranger. The supplement flatly limits trials to the period you indicate, although in practice most physicians will treat that as a guide rather than as an instruction.

If you initial Section 7 E be sure to fill in a number in the space to the left of "days"; otherwise you leave your agent exposed to pressure from physicians, your family, or any doubts of his own, to continue life-sustaining treatment longer than you would want. This is even more important in the supplement, since a physician who does not know you might interpret an empty space to mean that trials of life-sustaining treatment should continue until all possibilities have been exhausted.

Power of attorney at 8 (Supplement at 4), "My wishes concerning pain medications." Some life-threatening diseases and injuries cause severe pain. Pain impairs quality of life, and may even shorten duration of life (by making people stop eating; by impairing healing). But many physicians and nurses do not treat pain adequately. Doctors may not order enough medication, and nurses may give less than physicians prescribe.

Providers often mistrust patients' pain reports. Pain cannot be proved to be present, and cannot be measured. People who seem to be in the same physical condition often report very different levels of pain. Pain experience can depend on nonphysical factors, including uncertainty and fear about whether family and providers will accept a sick or injured person's decisions about medical care—especially physicians' and nurses' commitment to maintain comfort and alleviate pain. People whose pain is not treated effectively sometimes become irritable and demanding, which can make caregivers feel resentful, and even less responsive to pain information.

There is widespread lack of basic knowledge among providers about the amount, frequency, and manner of delivery of pain medications appropriate for effective pain relief. Often they inappropriately fear causing premature death or addiction.

Fear of premature death has to do with the fact that morphine—the primary medicine for severe pain—can depress breathing. Large enough amounts may stop breathing altogether, causing death. Morphine tolerance varies enormously from person to person, however, and people with severe pain often need, and can manage, huge amounts. Pain itself apparently creates tolerance. Also, tolerance increases as morphine is taken over time. Many physicians and nurses don't know this, and fall back on standard dosages instead of medicating each patient as needed.

People who receive even large amounts of morphine rarely become addicted. When they administer their medication themselves (a practice coming into wider use), they usually take only as much as they need. The various negative behavioral traits associated with drug addiction rarely occur with pain control in people who were not addicts already. When a person has severe discomfort (air insufficiency, for example) or pain that is expected to last for a long period of time or until death, medication dependence should not be of concern. A person who needs pain medication is no more an "addict" than someone who needs insulin, or any other medication, on a regular basis.

From the standpoint of concern for quality of life, undermedication is inappropriate not only medically, but also ethically. Physicians often give patients other potentially beneficial treatments that also carry a risk of death or other serious harm. They should not withhold pain control because they fear harm. Ethics statements of major physician organizations and the President's Commission for the Study of Ethical Problems in Medicine and Biomedical and Behavioral Research (in "Deciding to Forego Life-Sustaining Treatment") approve giving as much pain medication as appears to be needed for comfort, even if death results, as long as the intention is to give comfort rather than to cause death. (In Virginia, and implicitly in Washington, that principle is endorsed in law.)

"My wishes concerning pain medications" differs from Section 7 D treatment choices in a way that is important to providers, and important legally. Section 7 D authorizes your agent to refuse treatment you probably do not want. If you initial the first option in "My wishes concerning pain medications," you are requesting treatment you do want. A patient does not have a legal right to compel a physician to give treatment the physician considers damaging, and a provider who believes breathing failure or drug dependence might occur is not going to be convinced otherwise by a nonphysician. But, a physician or nurse who feels uneasy about these risks still might be willing to provide sufficient medication if she understands that *you* consider these risks less harmful than unrelieved pain. The purpose of this part is to tell your physicians and nurses what you want regarding pain medication, and to give them emotional permission to honor your wishes.

Be sure to discuss this part with your physician (and medical and nursing services directors if you are in or planning to enter a nursing home or other extended care facility) when you meet to talk about your health-care planning intentions and documents.

Power of attorney at 9 (Supplement at 5), "My wishes concerning pregnancy." Women who could possibly be pregnant when a health-care durable power of attorney might be implemented should say whether they want their wishes for withholding and withdrawing life-sustaining treatment expressed in Section 7 to apply during pregnancy.

Some health-care providers assume that any pregnant woman would want her life sustained if that would enable a child to be born. Also, as discussed in Chapter 1, many state laws provide that health-care planning documents do not apply during pregnancy,

and while such limitations are probably invalid, many providers may mistakenly believe that pregnant women must receive life-sustaining treatment. If you might be pregnant when your health-care planning document could become effective, and you would want life-sustaining treatment to be withheld and withdrawn just as if you were *not* pregnant, you need to discuss that with your provider and agents early on. Early discussion with your physician is particularly important because if for any reason he feels he cannot accept your intention, then you still have the option of changing physicians.

If you complete a state health-care planning form that contains a pregnancy exclusion you do not want, cross it out.

Note that Section 9 refers to trying to keep you alive for a fetus to mature sufficiently to be born "healthy." The word "healthy" implies that if prenatal testing were to show significant fetal impairment, your life should not be sustained to continue the pregnancy. The model documents are not intended to tell you what your choice should be. As with the rest of the document, if the pregnancy provision does not read as you intend then you should change it.

Power of attorney at 10 (Supplement at 6), "My wishes concerning other matters." Sometimes people want medical procedures that might help them but are experimental. Also, some people want to consent to autopsy, donation of organs and other body tissues, and/or donation of their remains for medical teaching and research. And, sometimes people want to give instructions for disposition of their remains in their durable power of attorney.

If you want your agent to have authority to consent to any of these, you should indicate that. Your agent might already have sufficient authority under Sections 1 and 4, and he certainly does in some states by law, but he might not know what you would want. Also, this expression of your wishes might head off opposition from your family.

Requesting, and consenting to, medical procedures that are experimental. A test or treatment is considered experimental if its effectiveness and safety for a particular condition have not yet been established. Sometimes there are no accepted tests or treatments for a condition. Or, the effectiveness of a treatment might be well known, but for some condition other than the one the patient has. Occasionally, preliminary testing of an unapproved test or treatment shows it to be so much more effective than the conventional practice that not to offer it seems wrong. In any of these circumstances experimental testing and treatment might be available.

When an experimental test or treatment is allowed to be used it is usually available only through certain medical centers or physicians. If your physician were to see you as a potential candidate for an experimental measure, she might offer referral to such a center or physician. Of course, you or your agent could also ask her about that.

As with any other treatment, whether you *want* experimental testing or treatment is a separate question from whether a physician is willing to *offer* it. Your agents and physician need to know whether you would want experimental testing and treatment if they might benefit you.

Autopsy. Autopsy is surgical opening of the body and examination of organs after death. The medical purpose is to learn something about a deceased person's injury or disease process that might help other people. It can require removing one or more organs, but is not disfiguring. If autopsy is indicated a physician will ask your agent, so your agent needs to know whether you would permit it.

Autopsy may be required by law if homicide or suicide has occurred or is suspected, or if death has been sudden and unexpected. If the law requires autopsy, it will be done whether or not the deceased person or his agent has approved.

Donation of organs and other tissue means transfer of those from a person who has died to a living person, or to several living people. Any competent adult can decide to be a donor. (If you are a minor, donation usually requires parental or guardian consent. If for some reason that is not feasible and you want to be able to donate, consult your physician, an organ donation organization such as the National Kidney Foundation, or an attorney.) Currently, various organs and tissues are transplanted routinely: heart, lungs, kidneys, liver, pancreas, corneas, skin, cartilage, bone, and bone marrow. Whether any of your organs or tissues may be suitable for transfer, and if so which ones, depends on various medical considerations that a physician can explain to you. Removal of organs for donation does not cause disfigurement.

Organs and other tissues are transplanted to save the lives of people who receive them, or to significantly improve the quality of their lives. Every year thousands of people who could be saved by organ or other tissue donation die because not enough transfer material is available. One reason for unavailability is that health-care providers often feel unable to ask permission from relatives whose loved one is about to die or has just died. When providers do ask, family members sometimes object because they are upset or angry, because they personally would not want to donate, or because they do not know what their loved one would have wanted. Giving permission in a health-care planning document, and talking with your family, can smooth the way for all concerned.

Medical teaching and research. Sometimes a body, or part of a body, is suitable for medical research or for teaching physicians in training. Body material—sometimes even just some cells—can be crucial to development of new medicines and medical techniques. Often remains can be respectfully buried or cremated when use for them has ended. If you would want your remains to be used for medical research or teaching, your agent needs to know that. Try to determine in advance whether your gift can be accepted.

Disposition of remains. Many people have particular wishes about what they want, or do not want, done with their bodies after death. They may want to be buried in a particular location, or to be cremated and have their ashes put or scattered in a certain place. Often people have wishes regarding religious services, and other matters.

It is best to leave such instructions in a property will, which clearly is valid after death, because legal authority of a health-care planning document after death, at least for disposition of remains, is currently uncertain in most states. If you do not have a will, or have not addressed disposition of remains in your will and you have particular wishes regarding disposition, you can describe them here and authorize your agent to carry them out.

If you have provided for disposition of remains in a will, you do not need to repeat them in your durable power of attorney. If you choose to do so, be sure that the instruc-

tions in the two documents are identical, and that the same person has the responsibility for implementing the instructions in both documents. If your wishes about disposition or your choice of personal representative (sometimes called "executor" or "administrator") have changed since you made your will, amend the will. Do not try to change instructions already in your will by saying something different in your power of attorney; that will only cause confusion and may result in your wishes not being followed. If your wishes have changed, change your will.

In the space at the end of Section 10, you can explain any wishes you might have regarding health care that have not been expressed anywhere else in the document. Some people feel strongly that they want to die at home, or in their nursing home or hospice, but not in a hospital. Other people want to avoid going to any nursing home, or want to indicate a particular choice of hospital or nursing home. Still others want their savings to be kept for their heirs rather than spent for prolonged treatment. (If you feel this way, it is very important for you to say so; most people automatically think the worst of an heir who says that a sick relative would want life-sustaining treatment stopped because of the cost.) Other matters may be important to you. If so, you should communicate them here.

Do not use this space, or any other part of your documents, to ask a physician to end your life or to give you the means to end your life. You would risk your entire document being effectively nullified, since many people believe consideration of suicide indicates at least possible mental instability. Also, assisting suicide is a serious crime in most states. A physician who knows you very well may be able to help you in a situation in which you are considering suicide, but only privately, not through documents. (Assisted suicide issues are outside the scope of this book. If you have a question about the legality of assisted suicide in your state, contact the Hemlock Society [P.O. Box 11830, Eugene, Oregon 97440, telephone 503–342–5748] and/or consult an attorney.)

If you are seriously considering suicide because of poor health and cannot discuss that with a physician, think about meeting with a thoughtful and skilled therapist to explore your reasons and options. Choose the therapist carefully; admitted suicidal intentions can lead to involuntary hospitalization for psychiatric observation and treatment. For help identifying therapists who will not do that, consider contacting a local support organization for people with serious illnesses, a clergy person, or the Hemlock Society.

Power of attorney at 11, "My wishes concerning guardianship." Every state has laws that provide for court appointment of a person to exercise legal authority for someone else who the court has determined cannot manage own personal and/or financial affairs. In most states such a person is called a "guardian" or "conservator," but a few states use other terms. Some state laws allow a judge to name a guardian only for personal care decisions or only to manage finances, but often one person is given complete authority to make both financial and personal decisions.

State laws allow a guardian or conservator to be appointed even if a person alleged to be incompetent has appointed an agent by a durable power of attorney. The law does that for two reasons. The first reason is to provide a way to question whether a particular durable power of attorney is valid. For example, the court would hear claims that an impaired person was pressured into appointing an agent, or did not understand what he was doing when he made his durable power of attorney. The second reason is to question whether an agent's decision is consistent with the intentions of the person who made it, or if those are not known, with the maker's best interests.

Guardianship actions involving health-care issues are usually brought by family members or health-care providers (an agent should not initiate guardianship proceedings unless health-care providers refuse to accept her authority), for one of two reasons: to choose a decision maker, or to replace one they believe is acting against the patient's wishes or best interest. Naming an agent by a durable power of attorney takes care of the first problem, but not the second.

If guardianship proceedings are brought, and the judge decides a guardian should be appointed but names someone other than your agent, your entire purpose in making a durable power of attorney could be defeated. For that reason the model document asks that if a guardian is appointed, your agent (or alternate) be the guardian.

You might wonder why, if a judge agrees that you need a guardian, she would appoint your agent. That can happen because if someone formally asks that a guardian be appointed and the judge finds you cannot make your own health-care decisions, the law might *require* that a guardian be named. If so, the judge might feel that the person you trust to be your agent would be the best choice. In some states the law requires that if a guardian is needed the agent be appointed, unless the judge finds that the agent is unfit.

If a judge appoints a guardian other than your agent or alternate, the durable power of attorney asks the judge to require the guardian to consult with the agent, and to act in accord with your values and intentions stated in your durable power of attorney. The judge is not bound to honor that request, but might do so. Even if she does not, the guardian might choose to honor your intentions by consulting your agent.

Power of attorney at 12 (Supplement at 7), "Protection of third parties who rely on my agent." The purpose of this section is to give health-care providers peace of mind that if they do their best to honor your wishes as expressed by your agent, they will not be liable for damages if someone (for example, an angry relative) sues them.

Power of attorney at 13 (Supplement at 8), "Revocation." The purposes of the first sentence of this section are to tell all concerned that: (1) you have a right to revoke your document; (2) you know you have that right; and (3) revocation can be accomplished in any way that gets the point across.

Be aware that if you revoke a document without replacing it with a new one, some people might interpret that to mean that you want all possible life-sustaining treatment (even though the law in many states says such interpretation is improper). If you want to revoke a document, but do not want maximum life-sustaining treatment, it is important to explain just what you do want to your providers, agents, and family.

You can revoke part of a document without revoking all of it, but if you do that you need to communicate clearly what is revoked and what is preserved. It is better to make a whole new document.

Illness can cause mental debilitation, during which people sometimes say or do things that seem inconsistent with treatment values expressed in a durable power of attorney, and/or seem to conflict with a decision of an agent. People are entitled to change their minds, but problems can arise when a physician and agent can't tell whether a person really has had a change of mind. It is unlikely that life-sustaining treatment would be withheld or withdrawn against a person's apparent current wishes, no matter what his mental status. The purpose of the second sentence of this section to convey that *if* an incapacitated person seems to contradict part of her durable power of attorney, or seems to disagree with a decision of her agent, that does not revoke her power of attorney in other respects or revoke her agent's authority.

Power of attorney at 14 (Supplement at 9), "Administrative provisions." This section addresses potentially important legal items.

a. Revocation of prior durable powers of attorney. This explains that the most recent document replaces all earlier ones. If you make a new document that differs significantly from earlier ones, you don't want confusion about which applies.

b. Interstate validity. Whether your durable power of attorney will be accepted in another state may depend on what the law there says about the particular health-care decision to be made. This section expresses your *intention* that your document be honored wherever it is presented.

c. Agent compensation. This directs that your agent not be paid for acting for you. Payment for serving as an agent could give rise to real or apparent conflicts of interest, and so should be avoided.

d. Agent financial responsibility. Your agent does not become financially responsible for your bills just by acting for you. But, he needs to be aware that he could *become* personally responsible if he accepts personal responsibility. When a person is admitted to a health-care facility, the admitting form will ask who is financially responsible for the patient. Your agent should not say he is, unless he is responsible for some reason other than being your agent (for example, a spouse in a state where the law makes spouses responsible for each other's health-care costs). If your agent is not financially responsible, he should give the provider your name, or the name of your health insurer (Medicare, private insurer, etc.).

e. When part of a legal document is determined to be legally invalid there can be a question about how much of the remainder should continue in effect. This provision says that if any part of your document is invalid (remember that the law pertaining to medical treatment issues is uncertain, and changing), you want the rest to be honored.

Power of attorney at 15 (Supplement at 10), "Summary." This part summarizes your intentions in making your document: to authorize an agent of your choice to make health-care decisions for you if you become unable make them personally, and, specifically, to authorize your agent to direct that life-sustaining treatment not be started, or be stopped.

Signing, witnessing, and notarization. It is extremely important that your documents meet the requirements of your state's laws for signature, and witnessing and/or notarization; deficiencies can result in their failing to qualify as legal documents. All legal requirements are listed in Chapter 6, Tables 1 and 2, and the related notes that follow the tables. (A document that is not formally legal should still have moral influ-

ence with your physician, and should also have some legal effect as evidence of your wishes, but you cannot count on these.)

Some states have special witness requirements for people who are patients or residents in health-care facilities, or who have applied for admission to such facilities, to assure that documents are made voluntarily and with understanding. These requirements appear in the notes after Tables 1 and 2.

Almost every state that requires witnessing excludes certain people from being witnesses. All restrictions are listed in Tables 1 and 2 and the notes after those tables.

When you choose witnesses, it is a good idea to avoid not only people who are disqualified when a document is signed, but also anyone who might be on your state's list of excluded people later on, when a document might be implemented. Some state laws make clear that witness exclusions matter only when a document is signed, not when it is implemented, but other laws are vague. As a result, providers can be confused. For example, if your spouse witnessed your document before you and she married, a physician who does not know you might not accept your document promptly because spouses cannot be witnesses. Such problems can be worked out, but you don't want them to crop up at a time when other matters are much more important.

All witness restrictions from nearly every state are included in Statement of Witnesses in the model documents. This makes the models easier for readers in most states to use, but it does not mean that every listed exclusion applies in every state. Also, in very few states an additional limitation might apply. It is a good idea that every witness exclusion in your state's law be mentioned in the Statement of Witnesses. If your state law excludes someone whom the Statement of Witnesses does not mention, you can insert that exclusion by hand; or, if some exclusion in the Statement of Witnesses is not required in your state and is inconvenient for you, you can draw a line through it. In either case, have your witnesses and a notary public if you use one put their initials after any insertion or deletion.

The Statement of Witnesses says in part that you signed your document in your witnesses' presence. If someone else signs for you because you are unable to do so, the statement needs to be modified. To do that, cross out "He/she signed this document in my presence," and substitute a statement that follows this example: "He said, in my presence, that this is his document but he is physically unable to sign it personally. He asked Bob Smith to sign his name for him, and Bob Smith did so in my presence." If the document is notarized, the notary statement will need to be modified similarly.

Even if your state does not require notar-ization, it can be useful if a question arises later about whether the signature on a document is yours, you appeared to sign voluntarily, deletions and additions were made when the document was signed, or the witnesses actually saw you sign. Also, in a few states, notarization can make up for witnessing by a disqualified witness. Finally, notarization can be essential if a document is being signed for a person who is physically unable to sign personally.

Notaries can be found in county and other local government offices, banks, savings and loans, realtors' offices, lawyers' offices, many health-care facilities, and elsewhere. If necessary, arrangements usually can be made for a notary to come to a house or health-care facility.

In Mississippi, in addition to other requirements declarations must be filed with the "bureau of vital statistics of the state board of health." The law does not say who has the responsibility to file, or how filing is to be done. Any health-care provider should be able to tell you how to do that.

CHAPTER 6

State Law Summaries

This chapter has a narrower focus than the previous chapters. It addresses each state's specific legal requirements for health-care planning documents. There are three tables and related notes. Table 1 covers requirements for health-care durable powers of attorney. Table 2 focuses on requirements for living wills and the supplement (Appendix B). Table 2 includes information about which states authorize implementing directives and declarations in the event of permanent unconsciousness, if your document says to do that. (Table 1 does not address unconsciousness regarding powers of attorney because an agent's authority to make decisions does not depend on a terminal condition or permanent unconsciousness, except in Nebraska, Ohio, Utah, and perhaps Tennessee.) Table 3 lists pregnancy restrictions.

You do not need to read the entire tables; just look at the information for the state or states that concern you.

As you read this chapter, please keep these points in mind:

- In every state (except Arizona, New Jersey, and in some circumstances Hawaii) the laws authorizing living wills provide that they apply only in the event of a terminal condition (or permanent unconsciousness, where noted in Table 2). Most living will laws, and a few power of attorney laws, say they do not apply during pregnancy. Some laws say they do not apply to certain treatments. It is important for you to know that both legally and practically you should be able to avoid those limitations, by using good documents and ensuring that your physician understands and accepts your choices.

- The requirements in Tables 1 and 2 (including the notes) must be satisfied for your documents to have full legal effect.

- The law can and does change. It is highly unlikely that a change would invalidate a document made under current law. But, many laws are limiting or confusing in important respects that new legislation can improve. If you learn of an important legal change, be sure to mention it to your physician; she might not know about it.

- No book substitutes for personal legal advice. If you have questions, consult a knowledgeable attorney in your own state.

INTRODUCTION TO TABLES 1 AND 2

In nearly every state, the laws that authorize health-care planning documents require signing, dating, and witnessing and/or notarization. In addition, health-care durable powers of attorney must name an agent.

State requirements on these points appear in Tables 1 and 2. Both tables are used the same way. Find the state that concerns you, then note the symbols on that state's line. Each symbol (except asterisks) is explained in the key that follows the table. Asterisks refer to information in the notes that follow the key after each table.

The keys for Tables 1 and 2 look very similar but are not identical. So, be sure to use the Table 1 key for Table 1, and the Table 2 key for Table 2.

Some of the states that are listed in Table 1 as not having health-care power of attorney laws provide for naming agents in declaration or directive forms. They are Arkansas, Louisiana, Minnesota, and Oklahoma. There, if you use the model health-care power of attorney in Appendix A, you should satisfy the requirements in Table 2.

Table 1. Legal Requirements for Health Care Durable Powers of Attorney (as of December 31, 1992)

	Signature Requirements	Agent Exclusions	Verification Requirements	Witness Exclusions	Disclosure Notices	Form Requirements
Alabama	(No health care power of attorney law.)					
Alaska	a		b			
Arizona	b		c	(b)^1,c^1,d*,e*,g,*		
Arkansas	(No health care power of attorney law.)					
California	b	(a)*	c*	(b)^1,c^1,(e)*,g	x	(x)
Colorado*						
Connecticut	a	a,*	a*	g		
Delaware	b		a*	b,(c),e,f		
D.C.	b		a	(b)^1,c^1,d,e		
Florida	b		a	b^1,g		
Georgia	b	a,b	a*			
Hawaii	b	a	d	(b),d,e		
Idaho	a	a*	c	b^1,g,*		
Illinois	a	a,b	*			
Indiana	b		d*		x	
Iowa	b	(a)	c	(b)^1,d,e*,g		
Kansas	a	(a)*,b	c	(b),c,f,g		(x)
Kentucky	b	*	c*	e*		
Louisiana	(No health care power of attorney law.)					

(continued)

Table 1. (*Continued*)

	Signature Requirements	Agent Exclusions	Verification Requirements	Witness Exclusions	Disclosure Notices	Form Requirements
Maine	a		c*			
Maryland	(No health care power of attorney law.)					
Massachusetts	b	b*	a	g		
Michigan	a	*	a	(b)*,c,d*,e,g		
Minnesota	(No health care power of attorney law.)					
Mississippi	a	(a)	c	(b)[1],c[1],d,(e),g	x	
Missouri	a	(a)*,b*	b			
Montana	b		a			
Nebraska	a	(a)*,b*	a*	(b)*,c,d*,g		(x)
Nevada	a	(a),b	c	(b)[1],c[1],d*,(e),g	x	(x)
New Hampshire	b	a*,b*	d	b*,c,d[1],e[1],g	x	(x)
New Jersey	b	b*	c	g		
New Mexico	b		a			
New York	b	a*,b*	a*	g		
North Carolina	a	a,b	d	(b)*,(c),d,e		
North Dakota	a	(a)*,b*	a	(b)*,(c),d,e,g	x	(x)
Ohio	a	(a)*,b*	c	(b),d*,g	x	
Oklahoma	(No health care power of attorney law.)					
Oregon	a	(a)*,b*	a	(b)[1],c[1],d*,g	x	x
Pennsylvania*						
Rhode Island	b	(a)*	a	(b)[1],c[1],d,(e),g	x	x
South Carolina	b	(a)*	d	(b),(c)*,d,e[1],f,g	x	(x)
South Dakota*						
Tennessee	a	(a)*,b*	d	(b)[1],(c)[1],d*,(e),g	x	
Texas	b	a*,b*	a	b*,(c),d,e,g	x	(x)
Utah*	a		b			(x)
Vermont	b	a*,b*	a*	b*,(c),d,e,g	x	(x)
Virginia	a		a	b		

(continued)

Table 1. (*Continued*)

	Signature Requirements	Agent Exclusions	Verification Requirements	Witness Exclusions	Disclosure Notices	Form Requirements
Washington	a	a*,b*	d*	b,(c),d,e		
West Virginia	b	a*,b*	d	a,b,c,d*,f,g		(x)
Wisconsin	b	a*,b*	a	(b),(c),(d)*,(e)*, f,g	x	(x)
Wyoming	b	a,b*	c	(b)^1,c^1,d,(e)*,g		

Key to Table 1:

1. *Signing requirements.* In all states, your document must be signed and dated.

    a. *You* must sign and date your document.

    b. Your document can be signed and dated by someone else for you, at your direction, if you are physically unable to do so.

2. *Agent exclusions.* In all states, your document must name an agent; naming an alternate is optional. The following people *cannot* be your agent or alternate:

    a. Your health-care provider (or, if the a is in parentheses, any of your provider's employees).

    b. An operator, administrator, or employee of any health-care facility where you are a patient or resident (including a physician if he is a facility employee).

3. *Verification requirements.* In all states, your document, including any pages you add to any form, must be witnessed and/or notarized.

    a. Witnessing is required, but not notarization.

    b. Notarization is required, but not witnessing.

    c. Either witnessing or notarization is required; the choice is yours.

    d. Both witnessing and notarization are required.

4. *Witness exclusions.* These people *cannot* be witnesses:

    a. Anyone who signs and dates your document for you at your request.

    b. Anyone related to you by blood or marriage (or, if the b is in parentheses, by adoption).

    c. Anyone entitled to any of your property when you die (and, if the c is in parentheses, anyone who might be owed money by your estate, such as a physician).

    d. Your attending physician or any employee of your attending physician.

    e. An operator of a health-care facility where you receive care, or an employee of such a facility, including a physician (and, if the e is in parentheses, an operator, administrator, or employee of *any* health-care facility, even if you do not receive care there).

    f. Anyone financially responsible for your medical care.

    g. Your agent or alternate agent named in a health-care durable power of attorney, or named in a declaration or directive in states where the law authorizes that.

    A 1 next to a letter in the "Witness exclusions" column means that one witness must not have that characteristic, but a second witness can have it.

5. If an X appears in this space, your state requires that a certain notice explaining the nature of health-care powers of attorney accompany whatever form you use. Such notices are already included in the power of attorney forms in Appendix D, except for Mississippi, Ohio, Tennessee and Vermont. Those states do not have a power of attorney form, but require that a "notice" or "warning" (which appears in Appendix D) accompany whatever form you use.

6. If an X appears in this space, you must use the specific power of attorney form in Appendix D. If

the X is in parentheses, that form is not required but you are strongly advised to use it.

Notes:

Arizona. Also excluded from witnessing is any person directly involved in providing health care to you (for example, a friend providing home care) when your document is witnessed. This exclusion applies as well to a notary, who also cannot be your agent. Only one witness is required.

California. Also excluded from being your agent is a nonrelative employee of your health-care provider; an operator of a community care facility or a residential care facility for the elderly; a nonrelative employee of such a facility. If you have a conservator, she cannot be your agent unless certain legal requirements are met, which require consulting a lawyer.

Also excluded from witnessing is any health-care provider and provider's employees, including any operator or employee of a community care facility or residential care facility for the elderly.

If you reside in a skilled nursing facility when you sign your durable power of attorney, a patient advocate or ombudsman authorized by the State Department of Aging must be one of the witnesses. That person must sign on one of the witness lines, and sign an additional statement that appears at the end of the state form.

Colorado. The law does not state any requirements for document validity. See the requirements for declarations in Table 2.

Connecticut. Also excluded from being your agent are operators and employees of a hospital, "home for the aged, rest home with nursing supervision, or chronic or convalescent nursing home" if you are a patient or resident when you sign your document, or if you have applied for admission. If you reside in such a facility, an administrator or employee of a government agency that is financially responsible for your medical care cannot be your agent unless related to you.

Witnesses for someone who resides in a facility operated or licensed by the state department of mental health must include at least one person who is a physician or clinical psychologist with specialized training in treating mental illness.

Witnesses for a person who resides in a facility operated or licensed by the department of mental retardation must include a least one witness who is a physician or clinical psychologist with specialized training in developmental disability.

Delaware. If you reside in any kind of nursing home when your power of attorney is signed, one of the two witnesses must be "a person designated as a patient advocate or ombudsman by either the Division of Aging or the Public Guardian." Neither of these people can have any of the characteristics that would exclude other witnesses.

Georgia. If you are a patient in a hospital or skilled nursing facility when your power of attorney is signed, your attending physician must witness it in addition to the other two witnesses.

Idaho. Also excluded from being your agent is an operator of a community care facility, a nonrelative employee of such a facility, or a nonrelative employee of any of your health-care providers.

Also excluded from witnessing are a community care facility operator, and employees of such a facility and of your health-care providers even if they are your relatives.

Illinois. Neither witnessing nor notarization is required. The form in the statute, which is optional, includes a space for one witness. For that reason, witnessing by at least one witness is strongly advised. See Table 2 for restrictions.

Indiana. The law contains conflicting verification requirements. Notarization and witnessing by at least one witness are strongly advised. See Table 2 for restrictions.

Iowa. Your health-care providers' employees can be witnesses if they are your relatives.

Kansas. A provider or his employee can be your agent if related to you, or if you and the agent are "members of the same community of persons who are bound by vows to a religious life and who conduct or assist in the conduct of religious service and actually and regularly engage in religious, benevolent, charitable or educational ministrations or the performance of health-care services."

Kentucky. Neither your agent, your witnesses, nor your notary public can be an owner, director, officer, or employee of a health-care facility where you are a patient or resident, unless related to you.

Maine. Applicable laws contain conflicting verification requirements. Notarization and witnessing are strongly advised. See Table 2 for witness restrictions.

Massachusetts. Also excluded from being your agent is an operator, administrator, or employee of a health-care facility where you are a patient or resident or have applied for admission.

Michigan. Before acting for you, your agent must sign the Michigan acceptance form in Appendix D.

Relatives excluded from witnessing are your spouse, parents, children, grandchildren, and siblings. Also excluded from witnessing are employees of a life or health insurance company that insures you. Employees of your physician are not excluded if they are not also employees of a facility where you are a patient or resident.

Missouri. See the Kansas note above.

Nebraska. An employee of your physician, or the owner, operator, or employee of a facility in which you are a patient or resident, can be your agent if related to you. A person who already is the agent for at least 10 people is excluded.

Witnesses must be at least 19 years old. Regarding witness exclusions, see the comments in the Michigan note. Also, only one witness may be an administrator or employee of your health-care providers.

Nevada. All physicians and their employees are excluded even if not involved in your care.

New Hampshire. Your residential care provider cannot be your agent. Your providers' employees are not excluded if related to you.

Your spouse is the only relative excluded from witnessing. One witness can be your health or residential care provider or provider's employee.

Whether notarization is required is unclear, so it is strongly advised.

New Jersey. This exclusion does not apply to a physician who is not involved in your care while acting as your agent. Also, any of these people can be your agent if related to you.

New York. Unless related to you, a physician, or an operator, administrator, or employee of a hospital is excluded from being your agent not only if you are a patient or resident, but also if you have applied for admission. Also, a doctor cannot act as your attending physician and agent at the same time. A person who, when your document is signed, is already the named agent for at least 10 people, cannot be your agent unless he is your spouse, child, parent, sibling, or grandparent, or is married to one of those relatives.

Witnesses to a health-care power of attorney for a person who resides in a facility operated or licensed by the state office of mental health must include at least one person not affiliated with the facility, and at least one physician certified by the American Board of Psychiatry and Neurology.

Witnesses to a health-care power of attorney for a person who resides in a facility operated or licensed by the office of mental retardation and developmental disability must include at least one person not affiliated with the facility, and at least one witness must be a physician or clinical psychologist who (1) is employed by a school for the retarded or disabled, (2) has been employed a minimum of two years to render care and service in a facility operated by the office of mental retardation and developmental disabilities, or (3) has been approved by the commissioner of mental retardation and developmental disabilities.

A superior court clerk or assistant clerk can certify your document instead of a notary public.

North Carolina. Also excluded are relatives of your spouse.

North Dakota. Agent exclusions do not apply to employees who are your relatives. Witnesses can include relatives by marriage.

Ohio. These agent exclusions do not apply to relatives or to fellow members of a religious order. Witnesses can include employees of your physician. An administrator of a nursing home where you receive care cannot be a witness.

Oregon. These people are not excluded from being your agent if related to you. Your physician's employees can be witnesses.

Pennsylvania. See the Colorado note.

Rhode Island. Also excluded from being your agent is an operator of a community care facility, and its employees not related to you. Nonrelative employees of your physician can be your agent. All health-care providers, operators of community care facilities, and their employees, are excluded from witnessing, even if related to you.

South Carolina. Also excluded from being your agent, unless related to you, is an employee of a nursing care facility in which you reside, and a spouse of any of your health-care providers or their employees. Also excluded from witnessing are beneficiaries of any life insurance you may have.

South Dakota. The law does not state any requirements for document validity. See the requirements for declarations in Table 2.

Tennessee. Your agent can be an employee of your provider or of a health-care institution, if related to you. If you have a conservator whom you want to be your agent, you need to consult an attorney. Excluded from witnessing are all health-care providers and their employees, even if not involved in your care.

Texas. An employee is not excluded from being your agent if related to you. The only relative automatically excluded from witnessing is a spouse. Be sure to sign your name on the line at the end of the disclosure statement in the state form.

Utah. Utah law authorizes only a "special power of attorney," in which you can designate a person you choose to make a living will for you.

Vermont. See the Texas note. Also, if you are being admitted to or are a resident of a nursing or residential care home when you make your document, "an ombudsman, recognized member of the clergy, at-torney licensed to practice in this state, or other person as may be designated by the probate court for the county in which the facility is located" must "sign a statement affirming that he or she has explained the nature and effect of the durable power of attorney for health care to [you]." If you are a patient or being admitted to a hospital when your health-care power of attorney is signed, "a person designated by the hospital" must "sign a statement that he or she has explained the nature and effect of the durable power of attorney for health care to [you]." A statement for either of those is included in the state form.

Be sure to sign the acknowledgment after the disclosure statement in the state form.

Washington. Any of these people can be your agent if he/she is your spouse, adult child, or sibling. The law is unclear about verification requirements, so both witnessing and notarization are recommended.

West Virginia. An employee is not excluded from being your agent if related to you. Also excluded from witnessing is a person who signs your document for you if you cannot do so. Your attending physician's employees can be witnesses.

Wisconsin. Also excluded from being your agent is the spouse of any of those people. Employees and spouses are not excluded if related to you. Your health-care providers and their employees when your document is made—except a chaplain or social worker—cannot be witnesses.

Wyoming. The agent and witness exclusions apply to operators and employees of community care and residential care facilities, but not other types of facilities.

Table 2. Legal Requirements for Declarations and Directives, Including the Supplement (as of December 31, 1992)

	Signature Requirements	Verification Requirements	Witness Exclusions	Permanent Unconsciousness
Alabama	b	a*	a,b,c,f	(x)
Alaska	b	b	b	
Arizona	b	b*	(b)[1],c[1],d*,e*,g	x
Arkansas	b	a		x
California	b	a*	c[1],d*,e*	x
Colorado	a	a	(c),d*,e*	
Connecticut	a	a		x
Delaware	b	a*	b,(c),e,f	
D.C.	b	a*	a,b,c,d,e,f	
Florida	b	a	b[1],g	x
Georgia	a	a*	b,(c),d,e,f	x
Hawaii	b	c	(b),d,e	x
Idaho	a	a		x
Illinois	b	a	a,c,f,*	
Indiana	b	a	a,(b)*,c,f	(x)
Iowa	b	b	(b)[1],d	x
Kansas	b	a	a,b,c,f	
Kentucky	b	a	c,d*,e,f	
Louisiana	a	a		x
Maine	b	a		x
Maryland	b	a	a,b,(c),f,*	
Massachusetts	(No law authorizing directives.)			
Michigan	(No law authorizing directives.)			
Minnesota	a	b	c,g	
Mississippi	a	a	b,(c),d	(x)
Missouri	b	a*	a	
Montana	b	a		

(continued)

Table 2. (*Continued*)

	Signature Requirements	Verification Requirements	Witness Exclusions	Permanent Unconsciousness
Nebraska	b	b*	e¹ *	x
Nevada	b	a		(x)
New Hampshire	a	c	b*,(c),d,e¹	x
New Jersey	b	b	g	x
New Mexico	b	a		x
New York	(No law authorizing directives.)			
North Carolina	a	c	b*,(c),d,e	x
North Dakota	b	a*	b,(c),d*,f	
Ohio	b	b	(b),d*,e*	x
Oklahoma	a	a	c	x
Oregon	a	a*	b,(c),d,e	
Pennsylvania	b	a	a	x
Rhode Island	b	a	b	(x)
South Carolina	a	c*	(b)*,(c)*,d,e¹,f	x
South Dakota	b	a		x
Tennessee	a	c	b,(c),d,e	x
Texas	a	a	b,(c),d,e*	
Utah	b	a	a,b,c,e,f	
Vermont	a	a	b*,(c),d	
Virginia	a	a	b	x
Washington	a	a	b,(c),d,e	x
West Virginia	b	c	a,b,c,d*,f,g	x
Wisconsin	b	a	(b),(c),(d)*,(e)*,f	x
Wyoming	b	a	a,b,c,f	

Key to Table 2:

1. *Signing requirements*. In all states, your document must be signed and dated.

    a. *You* must sign and date your document.

    b. Your document can be signed and dated by someone else for you, at your direction, if you are physically unable to do so.

2. *Verification requirements*. In all states, your document, including any pages you add to any form, must be witnessed and/or notarized.

a. Witnessing is required, but not notarization.

b. Witnessing or notarization is required; the choice is yours.

c. Both witnessing and notarization are required.

3. *Witness exclusions.* These people *cannot* be witnesses:

a. Anyone who signs and dates your document for you at your request.

b. Anyone related to you by blood or marriage (or, if the b is in parentheses, by adoption).

c. Anyone entitled to any of your property when you die (and, if the c is in parentheses, anyone who might be owed money by your estate, such as a physician).

d. Your attending physician or any employee of your attending physician.

e. An operator of a health-care facility where you receive care, or an employee of such a facility, including a physician (and, if the e is in parentheses an operator, administrator, or employee of any health-care facility, even if you do not receive care there).

f. Anyone financially responsible for your medical care.

g. Your agent or alternate agent named in a health-care durable power of attorney, or named in a declaration or directive in states where the law authorizes that.

A 1 next to a letter in the "Witness exclusions" column means that one witness must not have that characteristic, but a second witness can have it.

4. If an X appears in this space, the law defines "terminal condition" to include permanent unconsciousness, or otherwise expressly provides that a declaration or directive can be implemented in the event of permanent unconsciousness. If the X is in parentheses that is implied, not express.

Notes:

Alabama. Witnesses must be at least 19 years old.

Arizona. For witness rules, see Arizona note after Table 1.

California. If you reside in a skilled nursing facility or a long term care facility when you sign your declaration and the supplement, one of the two witnesses must be a patient advocate or ombudsman authorized by the state department of aging.

These are excluded from witnessing even if not involved in your care: any health-care provider, or operator of a community care facility, or residential care facility for the elderly, and their employees.

Colorado. Physicians are excluded even if not involved in your care. If you are a patient or resident in a health-care facility, other patients and residents are excluded.

Connecticut. Regarding witnessing, see Connecticut note after Table 1.

Delaware. Regarding a special witness requirement, see Delaware note after Table 1.

District of Columbia. If a person resides in an "intermediate care or skilled care facility" when his declaration is made, one of the two witnesses must be a "patient care advocate or ombudsman," with the same qualifications as other witnesses.

Georgia. If a person is a patient in a hospital or skilled nursing facility when her living will is made, a third witness is required, who must be either (1) in a hospital, the chief of the medical staff, and physician not involved in the patiet's care, or any staff person not involved in the patient's care and designated by the hospital administrator and chief of medical staff, or (2) in a nursing facility, the medical director or any staff physician not involved in the patient's care.

Illinois. Whether these exclusions are mandatory is unclear.

Indiana. Relatives excluded are your spouse, parents, and children.

Kentucky. Your attending physician's employees are not excluded unless they are also employees of a facility where you are a patient.

Maryland. See the Arizona note after Table 1 (but two witnesses are required). Also, a member of a law firm that has been designated as the personal representative under a property will cannot witness.

Missouri. Your document is not required to be witnessed if it is entirely in your handwriting and signed by you.

Nebraska. Witnesses must be at least 19 years old. No witness may be an employee of a life or health insurance company that insures you.

New Hampshire. The only relative automatically excluded from witnessing is your spouse. If you are a patient or resident of a health-care facility, only one witness may be that provider's employee.

North Carolina. Also excluded are relatives of your spouse.

North Dakota. If you reside in a long-term-care facility when you make your declaration, one of the witnesses must be "a recognized member of the clergy, an attorney licensed to practice in this state, or a person as may be designated by the department of human services or the county court for the county in which the facility is located." Your physicians' employees are not excluded from witnessing.

Ohio. Your physicians' employees are not excluded. The administrator of any nursing home in which you receive care is excluded.

Oregon. If you reside in a long-term-care facility when you make your document, one witness must be a person designated by the department of human resources.

South Carolina. If you are a hospital patient or nursing care facility resident when you make your document, one of your witnesses must be an ombudsman designated by the state ombudsman, office of the governor. The notary public may also be a witness. Also excluded from witnessing are spouses of any of your relatives, and beneficiaries of any life insurance you may have.

Tennessee. Whether notarization is required is unclear, so it is strongly recommended.

Texas. If you are a patient or resident in a health-care facility, other patients and residents are excluded.

Vermont. The only relative automatically excluded from witnessing is your spouse.

West Virginia. Your physicians' employees are not excluded.

Wisconsin. Regarding witnessing, see the Wisconsin note after Table 1.

Table 3. Pregnancy Restrictions (as of December 31, 1992)

Two types of pregnancy restriction appear in the laws:

A. Suspension of a document at any time during pregnancy.
B. Suspension during pregnancy if continuing life-sustaining treatment would enable the fetus to be born alive.

"L.W." means the type of pregnancy restriction indicated appears in a law that authorizes living will documents. "D.P.A." means the type of pregnancy restriction indicated appears in a law that authorizes health-care durable powers of attorney. An x in brackets in the D.P.A. column means that a pregnancy restriction appears in a living will law that authorizes naming an agent in that kind of document.

	L.W.	D.P.A.	Type
Alabama	x		A
Alaska	x		B
Arkansas	x	[x]	B
California	x		A
Colorado	x		B[1]
Connecticut	x		A
Delaware	x	[x]	A
Florida		x	A[2]
Georgia	x		B[3]
Hawaii	x		A
Idaho	x		B
Illinois	x		B
Indiana	x		A
Iowa	x		B
Kansas	x		A
Kentucky	x	x	A (L.W.); B (D.P.A.[4,5])
Maryland	x		A
Michigan	x		A
Minnesota	x	[x]	B
Mississippi	x		A
Missouri	x		A
Montana	x	[x]	B
Nebraska	x	x	B
Nevada	x		B
New Hampshire	x	x	A (L.W.); B (D.P.A.[4])
North Dakota	x		A
Ohio	x	x[6]	B
Oklahoma	x	[x]	A[5]
Pennsylvania	x		B[4]
Rhode Island	x		B
South Carolina	x	x	A
South Dakota	x	x	B[4]
Texas	x		A

(continued)

Table 3. (*Continued*)

	L.W.	D.P.A.	Type
Utah	x	x	A
Washington	x[7]		A
Wisconsin	x[8]		A
Wyoming	x		A

[1] Life-sustaining treatment may be withheld or withdrawn during pregnancy if the fetus is not viable.

[2] Life-sustaining treatment may be withheld or withdrawn if your document authorizes that during pregnancy.

[3] Life-sustaining treatment to be provided unless fetus is not viable and the document expressly provides that it is intended to apply during pregnancy.

[4] Life-sustaining treatment to be provided unless it would prolong severe pain that cannot be alleviated by pain medication, or would harm the pregnant woman in some other way.

[5] Before withholding or withdrawing life-sustaining treatment, a physician is supposed to test for pregnancy if pregnancy has not yet been diagnosed.

[6] Life-sustaining treatment to be provided unless that would put the woman's life at substantial risk, or the fetus would not be born alive.

[7] The pregnancy restriction appears only in the optional directive form, not in any mandatory part of the statute.

[8] The pregnancy restriction appears in the form, not elsewhere in the law, and whether that form must be used is unclear.

Durable Power of Attorney for Health-Care Decisions

1. When I want this power of attorney to be effective:

If I become unable to make my own health-care decisions because of illness or injury, I want all such decisions to be made for me by my health-care agent.

I understand that I might become unable to make decisions but then recover. I also understand that even when I cannot make a particular decision I still might be able to make others. When I can make my own decisions, I want to do so. When I cannot, I want my agent to make them for me.

I want my physician and my agent to be in agreement about whether I can or cannot make a decision. If they disagree, then my agent may have me examined by another physician, whose decision I want to be determinative.

Even if I cannot make a health-care decision, I want my physician and agent to talk to me honestly about my condition and treatment if they think I might be able to understand.

I want this document to apply whether or not I have a terminal condition when any question arises about whether to implement it, and no matter when my death is expected to occur.

If I make a written declaration or directive to physicians for health-care decisions, I want that to apply only if a health-care agent named in this power of attorney is not available when a health-care decision must be made.

I want this durable power of attorney to continue to operate after my death, for my agent to consent to autopsy, organ donation, use of my body for medical research, and disposition of my remains, if I authorize these in Section 10 below.

2. My health-care agent:

Name/Relationship: _____

Address: _____

Telephone: home (_____)_____ work (_____)_____

3. My alternate agent [optional]:

If my agent becomes unable or unwilling to serve; or is unavailable when needed; or if he/she is a spouse from whom I am separated; then I name this alternate:

Name/Relationship: _____

Address: _____

Telephone: home (_____)_____ work (_____)_____

If the reason the alternate acts for me is unavailability of my first agent, then I want the alternate to act only as long as the first agent is unavailable.

4. The authority I want my agent to have:

I grant my agent complete authority to make decisions about my health care. I want my agent to be able to exercise the broadest authority for health-care decision making that I have myself as a competent adult under the United States Constitution, any United States statute or case law, the common law, and the constitution, statutes, or case law of any state in which this document is presented.

I intend that my agent's powers include, but not be limited to: (a) consenting and refusing consent to any medical procedure recommended by my physicians, and withdrawing consent to any procedure already in use (even if started at my request or with my consent); (b) requesting particular medical procedures; (c) complete access to my medical records and information, including disclosure to others; (d) employing and dismissing health-care providers (binding me, or any insurer of mine, to pay for the same); (e) transferring me from any health-care facility, even against medical advice, to another facility, a private residence, or some other place; (f) taking any other action necessary to do what I authorize in this document.

5. How I want my agent to make decisions for me:

I want my agent to decide and act as he/she believes I would want in the circumstances. If my agent does not know what I would want, then I want him/her to decide and act as he/she believes is in my best interest, considering his/her knowledge of me, the contents of this document, and medical information provided by my physicians.

6. Why I am making this power of attorney:

I value life very much, but not life above all else. If I ever have a life-threatening condition and cannot make my own health-care decisions, I do not want to be given life-sustaining treatment automatically; I want decisions about use of such treatment to be made by my agent, guided by this document.

Whether to accept a treatment when offered, or to repeat or continue a treatment I accepted before, comes down to my personal choice. Effects of treatment that others might consider beneficial I might not. What others might consider a reasonable likelihood of benefit, justifying the probable or possible burdens of treatment, I might see differently. When I cannot express those choices personally I want my health-care agent to do that for me. I do not want others to substitute their choices for mine or my agent's because they think their knowledge or values are better, or because they think their choices are in my best interest. I do not want my intentions and judgments to be dismissed because someone thinks that if I had had more information when I made this document, or if I had known certain medical facts that developed later, I would change my mind. If I become unable to make health-care decisions personally, I want my physicians and family to honor my values, intentions, and judgments expressed here, as applied by my agent.

[You may make other values statements here if you wish. If the space is insufficient, write "see attachment" on the last line and continue on another page. If you do not want to add anything, put an X across the lines.]

_____

_____

_____

_____

7. My choices concerning life-sustaining treatment:
[Read all of Section 7 carefully before making any marks.]

_____ A.   I have lived a long life and I am ready to accept death when it comes. For that reason, if I become unable to make my own health-care decisions, and I have or get a life-threatening condition, I want no life-sustaining treatment, even if the reason for such treatment might be completely reversible.

_____ B.   Because of health losses I have experienced, I consider my quality of life to be unacceptable, or only marginally acceptable. For that reason, if I become unable to make my own health-care decisions, and I have or get a life-threatening condition, I want no life-sustaining treatment, even if the reason for such treatment might be completely reversible.

[*If you initial this statement, explain why here. If you need more space, write "see attachment" at the end of the space and continue on another page.*]

_____

_____

_____

_____

_____

STOP: If you initialed Statement A or B, cross out Part C; initial every treatment in Part D; and initial the second choice in Part E.

If you did not initial Statement A or B (put a dash in any space you did not initial), complete Section 7, Parts C through E now.

C.   My current quality of life is acceptable, but if my quality of life were to become very poor, and I were to have or get a life-threatening condition, then I would want to be allowed to die, while receiving only non-life-sustaining comfort care (unless I authorize temporary use of life-sustaining treatment later in this section).

These are the qualities of life I consider so poor that I would want to be allowed to die [*initial as you choose; put a dash in any space you do not initial*]:

_____ 1.   Unconsciousness (chronic coma or persistent vegetative state) from which ability to think and communicate probably will not be recovered, or, unconsciousness lasting [*insert number*] _____ days, whichever occurs first.

or

_____ 2.   Brain damage that probably is not reversible, and causes apparently complete, or nearly complete, loss of ability to think or communicate, but not loss of consciousness.

or

_____ 3.   Total physical dependence on others for care, because of deterioration that probably is not reversible.

or

_____ 4.   Pain control that is inadequate, either because pain cannot be eliminated, or because the amount of medicine needed to eliminate pain causes so much sedation that ability to communicate verbally is lost.

or

_____ 5.   [*If there are circumstances in which you would not want life-sustaining treatment besides any initialed above, initial the blank to the left of 5. and describe the circumstances here. If you need more space, write "see attachment" on the last line and continue on another page. If you do not want to add anything, put a dash in the space to the left of the 5. and an X across the lines.*]

_____

_____

_____

_____

_____

D.   Particular life-sustaining treatments.

If I initialed 7 A or B, I do not want any of these life-sustaining treatments to be started, and if already in use I want them stopped.

If I initialed any of 7 C, I do not want these life-sustaining treatments, unless I authorize temporary use in Part 7 E [*initial each treatment you want your agent to be able to refuse or stop; put a dash in any space you do not initial*]:

_____   Nutrition and hydration, other than ordinary food and water delivered by mouth, if I cannot eat and drink at all, or enough to sustain me.

_____   All cardiopulmonary resuscitation measures, to try to restart my heart and breathing if they stop.

_____   Mechanical ventilation (breathing by machine), if I cannot breathe adequately.

_____   Surgeries that would prolong my life.

_____   Dialysis or filtration, to clean life-threatening substances from my blood if my kidneys fail.

_____   Transfusion of blood or blood products, to replace lost or diseased blood.

_____   Medications, when their purpose is to treat life-threatening conditions rather than control pain (for example, antibiotics, chemotherapy, insulin).

_____   Anything else that sustains, restores or replaces a vital body function.

E.   Temporary use of life-sustaining treatment.

If I experience an unacceptable quality of life, and my physician believes that temporary use of life-sustaining treatment will restore me to health that I consider acceptable, then [*initial one, only; put a dash in the space you do not initial*]:

_____   My agent may consent to life-sustaining treatment, for a period not to exceed about _____ days.

_____   I still do not want life-sustaining treatment.

8.   *My wishes concerning pain medication:*

If I appear to be in pain I want enough medication to make me comfortable, even if my physician believes that might hasten my death or cause drug dependency [*initial one only; put a dash in the space you do not initial*]:

_____ Yes   _____ No

9.   *My wishes concerning pregnancy:*

If I experience a life-threatening condition during pregnancy, but I probably could be kept alive long enough for my fetus to mature sufficiently to be born healthy [*if this section could apply to you, initial one space and put a dash in the other space; if the section cannot apply to you, put an X across the whole section*]:

_____   I would want my life sustained to try to accomplish that.

_____   I would want decisions about life-sustaining treatment to be made as if I were not pregnant.

10.   *My wishes concerning other matters:*

I authorize my agent to [*initial as you choose; put a dash in any space you do not initial*]:

Yes   No

_____   _____   request, and consent to, medical procedures that are experimental

_____   _____   consent to autopsy

_____   _____   consent to donation of organs or other tissues

_____   _____   consent to donation of all or part of my body for medical teaching and research

_____   _____   dispose of my remains as follows [*If you initial this part, write your instructions to your agent on the lines provided; if you also have provided for disposition of remains in a will, do not do so here*]:

_____

_____

_____

[*If you want to state other kinds of choices, you can do that here. If you need more space, write "see attachment" on the last line and continue on another page. If you do not want to add anything, put an X across the lines.*]

_____

_____

_____

_____

11. *Guardianship:*

If a guardian is appointed for me, I want my health-care agent to be the guardian, or if he/she cannot serve, then I want my alternate. If the court decides to name someone else, I ask that the court require the guardian to consult with my agent (or alternate, if the alternate has been acting as my agent) concerning all health-care decisions that would require my consent if I were acting for myself, and require the guardian to act in accord with this document.

12. *Protection of third parties who rely on my agent:*

No person who in good faith relies on representations of my agent or alternate agent will be liable to me, my estate, my heirs, or my assigns, for accepting the agent's authority.

13. *Revocation:*

This durable power of attorney can be revoked by any oral or written statement by me to that effect, or by any other expression of my intention to revoke. If I express disagreement with a decision my agent makes, that disagreement, alone, is not a revocation.

14. *Administrative provisions:*

a. I revoke any prior health-care planning documents.

b. I intend that this power of attorney be valid in any state in which it is presented.

c. I intend that my agent not be entitled to compensation for services performed under this power of attorney.

d. I intend that my agent not be financially responsible for any expense related to my health care because of his/her status as my agent, or because of exercise of his/her agency authority, and, I want my agent to be reimbursed from any available source for all reasonable expenses incurred as a result of exercising powers granted by this document.

e. If any part of this document is legally determined to be invalid, I want the remainder to continue in effect.

15. *Summary:*

I understand what this document means: I am naming an agent to make health-care decisions for me if I become unable to make them myself. As provided above, I want my agent to direct that life-sustaining treatment not be started, and if already in use be stopped, even if that will result in my death occurring sooner than if everything medically possible were done. I make this document of my own free will. I have the mental and emotional capacity to do so.

DATED this _____ day of _____, 199_____.

_____   _____
Signature   Printed name

City, County, and State of Residence: _____

Statement of Witnesses:
Each of the undersigned witnesses affirms as follows:
_____ is personally known to me. He/she signed this document in my presence. I believe him/her to be of sound mind, and to have made this health-care durable power of attorney voluntarily, intentionally, and with understanding of its contents. I am at least 18 years old; not related to him/her by blood, adoption, or marriage; have no claim against his/her estate; am not directly financially responsible for his/her medical care; and am not an agent named in this document. He/she has stated that I am not a beneficiary of his/her will or any codicil. I certify under penalty of perjury under the law of this state that this *Statement Of Witnesses* is true.

_____   _____
Signature   Signature

_____   _____
Print name   Print name

Date: _____   Date: _____

Address: _____   Address: _____

_____   _____

Telephone: (_____)_____   Telephone: (_____)_____

Notarization:

STATE OF _____   )
) ss.
COUNTY OF _____   )

On this day, the person known to me to be _____ personally appeared before me and executed the preceding Durable Power of Attorney for Health-Care Decisions. He/she acknowledged that he/she signed the same voluntarily, for the purposes the instrument describes.

Also on this date, the witnesses named above witnessed the signing of the Durable Power of Attorney for Health-Care Decisions and signed the Statement of Witnesses before me.

GIVEN under my hand and official seal on _____.

_____
NOTARY PUBLIC in and for the State

of _____, residing at _____.

My commission expires: _____.

Supplement to Directive or Declaration to Physicians

1. When I want this document to be effective:

If I become unable to make my own health-care decisions because of illness or injury, and I have not made a health-care power of attorney naming an agent to make such decisions for me, then I want my physician to act, as provided in this document. If I have a health-care power of attorney, I want my agent to make those decisions, with my physician's advice.

I understand that I might become unable to make decisions but then recover. I also understand that even when I cannot make a particular decision I still might be able to make others. When I can make my own decisions, I want to do so.

Even if I cannot make a health-care decision, I want my physician to talk to me honestly about my condition and treatment if he/she thinks I might be able to understand.

I want this document to apply whether or not I have a terminal condition when any question arises about whether to implement it, and no matter when my death is expected to occur.

I want this document to be applied in a way that reflects the broadest rights for health-care decision making that I have as a competent adult under the United States Constitution, any United States statute or case law, the common law, and the constitution, statutes, and case law of any state in which this document is presented, as those rights exist now or as they might be expanded in the future. I intend that this document expand any attached directive or declaration, and not be restricted in any way by it or by any law in which it appears.

I want this document to continue to operate after my death, for my agent to consent to autopsy, organ donation, use of my body for medical research, and disposition of my remains, if I authorize those in Part 6 below.

2. Why I am making written instructions for my physicians:

I value life very much, but not life above all else. If I ever have a life-threatening condition and cannot make my own health-care decisions, I do not want to be given life-sustaining treatment automatically. I want decisions about use of such treatment to be made by my health-care agent, if I have made a durable power of attorney for health care. If I have not made a durable power of attorney, then I want decisions about use of life-sustaining treatment to be made for me as I provide in this document.

If I initial Part 3 A or B below, I do not want life-sustaining medical treatment at all; I want only non-life-sustaining comfort care. If my quality of life becomes unacceptable as initialed in 3 C, and I have or get a life-threatening condition, I do not want life-sustaining treatment, unless in part 3 E I authorize it for a limited period if it probably would restore me to a quality of life I consider acceptable. If I become unable to express these intentions personally, and I do not have a health-care agent, I intend that this document speak for me.

Whether to accept a treatment when offered, or to repeat or continue a treatment I accepted before, comes down to my personal choice. Effects of treatment that others might consider beneficial I might not. What others might consider a reasonable likelihood of benefit, justifying the probable or possible burdens of treatment, I might see differently. I do not want others to substitute their choices for mine or my agent's because they think their knowledge or values are better, or because they think their choices are in my best interest. I do not want my intentions and judgments to be dismissed because someone thinks that if I had had more information when I made this document, or if I had known certain medical facts that developed later, I would change my mind. If I become unable to make health-care decisions personally, I want my physicians and family to honor my values, intentions, and judgments expressed here.

[*You may make other values statements here if you wish. If the space is insufficient, start here, then write "see attachment" on the last line and continue on another page. If you don't want to add anything here, put an X across the space.*]

_____

_____

_____

_____

3. *My choices concerning life-sustaining treatment:*
    [*Read all of Section 3 carefully before making any marks.*]

_____ A.   I have lived a long life and I am ready to accept death when it comes. For that reason, if I become unable to make my own health-care decisions, and I have or get a life-threatening condition, I want no life-sustaining treatment, even if the reason for such treatment might be completely reversible.

_____ B.   Because of health losses I have experienced, I consider my quality of life to be unacceptable, or only marginally acceptable. For that reason, if I become unable to make my own health-care decisions, and I have or get a life-threatening condition, I want no life-sustaining treatment, even if the reason for such treatment might be completely reversible.

[*If you initial this statement, explain why here. If you need more space, write "see attachment" at the end of the space and continue on another page.*]

_____

_____

_____

_____

STOP: If you initialed statement A or B, cross out Part C; initial every treatment in Part D; and initial the second choice in Part E.

If you did not initial Statement A or B (put a dash in any space you did not initial), complete Section 3, Parts C through E now.

C.   My current quality of life is acceptable, but if my quality of life were to become very poor, and I were to have or get a life-threatening condition, then I would want to be allowed to die, while receiving only non-life-sustaining comfort care (unless I authorize temporary use of life-sustaining treatment later in this section).

These are the qualities of life I consider so poor that I would want to be allowed to die [*Initial as you choose; put a dash in any space you do not initial*]:

_____ 1.   Unconsciousness (chronic coma or persistent vegetative state) from which ability to think and communicate probably will not be recovered, or, unconsciousness lasting [*insert number*] _____ days, whichever occurs first.

or

_____ 2.   Brain damage that probably is not reversible, and causes apparently complete, or nearly complete, loss of ability to think or communicate, but not loss of consciousness.

or

_____ 3.   Total physical dependence on others for care, because of deterioration that probably is not reversible.

or

_____ 4.   Pain control that is inadequate, either because pain cannot be eliminated, or because the amount of medicine needed to eliminate pain causes so much sedation that ability to communicate verbally is lost.

or

_____ 5.   [*If there are circumstances in which you would not want life-sustaining treatment besides any initialed above, initial the blank to the left of 5. and describe the circumstances here. If you need more space, write "see attachment" on the last line and continue on another page. If you do not want to add anything, put a dash in the space to the left of the 5. and an X across the lines.*]

_____

_____

_____

_____

_____

D.   Particular life-sustaining treatments.

If I initialed 3 A or B, I do not want any of these life-sustaining treatments to be started, and if already in use I want them stopped.

If I initialed any of 3 C, I do not want these life-sustaining treatments, unless I authorize temporary use in Part 3 E [*initial each treatment you do not want; put a dash in any space you do not initial*]:

_____   Nutrition and hydration, other than ordinary food and water delivered by mouth, if I cannot eat and drink at all, or enough to sustain me.

_____   All cardiopulmonary resuscitation measures, to try to restart my heart and breathing if they stop.

_____   Mechanical ventilation (breathing by machine), if I cannot breathe adequately.

_____   Surgeries that would prolong my life.

_____ Dialysis or filtration, to clean life-threatening substances from my blood if my kidneys fail.

_____ Transfusion of blood or blood products, to replace lost or diseased blood.

_____ Medications, when their purpose is to treat life-threatening conditions rather than control pain (for example, antibiotics, chemotherapy, insulin).

_____ Anything else that sustains, restores, or replaces a vital body function.

E. Temporary use of life-sustaining treatment.

If I experience an unacceptable quality of life, and my physician believes that temporary use of life-sustaining treatment will restore me to health that I consider acceptable, then [_initial one, only; put a dash in the space you do not initial_]:

_____ My physician may use life-sustaining treatment, for a period not to exceed about _____ days.

_____ I still do not want life-sustaining treatment.

4. _My wishes concerning pain medication:_

If I appear to be in pain I want enough medication to make me comfortable, even if my physician believes that might hasten my death or cause drug dependency [_initial one only; put a dash in the space you do not initial_].

_____ Yes   _____ No

5. _My wishes concerning pregnancy:_

If I experience a life-threatening condition during pregnancy, but I probably could be kept alive long enough for my fetus to mature sufficiently to be born healthy [_if this section could apply to you, initial one space and put a dash in the other space; if the section cannot apply to you, put an X across the whole section_]:

_____ I would want my life sustained to try to accomplish that.

_____ I would want decisions about life-sustaining treatment to be made as if I were not pregnant.

6. _My wishes concerning other matters:_

[_Initial as you choose; put a dash in any space you do not initial._]

Yes	No	
_____	_____	I consent to medical procedures that are experimental and that my physician considers in my best interest, subject to my statements in preceding sections.
_____	_____	I consent to autopsy.
_____	_____	I consent to donation of organs or other tissues.
_____	_____	I consent to use of all or part of my body for medical teaching and research.

7. _Protection of third parties who rely on my agent:_

No person who in good faith relies on representations of my agent or alternate agent shall be liable to me, my estate, or my heirs or my assigns, for accepting the agent's authority.

8. _Revocation:_

This durable power of attorney can be revoked by any oral or written statement by me to that effect, or by any other expression of my intention to revoke. However, if I express disagreement with a decision my agent makes, that disagreement, alone, is not a revocation.

9. _Administrative provisions:_

I revoke any prior health-care planning documents.

If any part of this document is held unenforceable by a court, I intend that all other parts continue in force as I have expressed them.

I intend that this document be valid in any jurisdiction in which it is presented.

10. Summary:

I understand what this document means. If I become unable to make decisions about use of life-sustaining medical treatment, I intend that this document speak for me, and be honored by my family and my health-care providers (unless I have made a durable power of attorney for health care, in which case I want that document, and my agent's decisions, to control). I accept that my death would follow not starting, or stopping, life-sustaining treatment; I intend and ask that my family and providers accept that, too.

I make this document of my own free will. I have the mental and emotional capacity to do so.

Signed _____

Print name: _____

Residing in (city, county, and state) _____

Statement of Witnesses:

Each of the undersigned witnesses affirms as follows:

_____ is personally known to me. He/she signed this document in my presence. I believe him/her to be of sound mind, and to have made this Supplement to Directive or Declaration to Physicians voluntarily, intentionally, and with understanding of its contents. I am at least 18 years old; not related to him/her by blood, adoption, or marriage; have no claim against his/her estate at the time of execution of this document; am not directly financially responsible for his/her medical care; and not named as an agent in his/her health-care power of attorney. He/she has stated that I am not a beneficiary of his/her will or any codicil. I certify under penalty of perjury under the law of this state that this Statement of Witnesses is correct and true.

Witness: _____   Witness: _____

Print name: _____   Print name: _____

Address: _____   Address: _____

_____   _____

Telephone: _____   Telephone: _____

Notarization:

STATE OF _____   )
) ss.
COUNTY OF _____   )

On this day, the person known to me to be _____ personally appeared before me and executed the preceding Supplement to Directive or Declaration to Physicians. He/she acknowledged that he/she signed the same voluntarily, for the purposes the instrument describes.

Also on this date, the witnesses named above witnessed the signing of the Supplement to Directive or Declaration to Physicians and signed the Statement of Witnesses in my presence.

GIVEN under my hand and official seal on _____.

_____

NOTARY PUBLIC in and for the State
of _____, residing at _____.
My commission expires: _____.

Notice of Revocation of Health-Care Planning Document

I, _____, residing in (insert city, county, and state) _____, give notice that I revoke [initial one or both; put a dash in any space you do not initial]

_____ any durable power of attorney for health-care decisions
_____ any directive or declaration to physicians

dated before today's date: _____, 199_____.

_____   _____
Signature   Printed name

[Optional]

Witness: _____   Witness: _____

Print name: _____   Print name: _____

Address: _____   Address: _____

_____   _____

Telephone: _____   Telephone: _____

95

State Living Will, Power of Attorney, and Other Forms

This appendix contains the following, in alphabetical order by state:

1. the living will form for each state where the law includes one, and the District of Columbia
2. the power of attorney form for each state where the law requires use of the specific form, or a substantially similar form
3. "notices" for Mississippi, Ohio, and Wisconsin, and a "warning" for Tennessee, which must be attached to whatever health-care power of attorney you use in those states
4. an "addendum" that must be attached to a health-care power of attorney in Indiana
5. a form to revoke a declaration in Mississippi
6. a special definitions form that must be attached to Ohio documents that apply in the event of a "terminal condition" or "permanently unconscious state"
7. the agent's acceptance form for Michigan

Read the state living will and power of attorney forms especially carefully. Make sure that the choices you make in them are consistent with your choices in the model forms in Appendixes A and B. As with the model forms, put a dash in any space you do not initial or cross the space out.

INSTRUCTIONS FOR COORDINATING CERTAIN STATES' FORMS WITH THE MODEL DOCUMENTS

Arizona: If you make both a health-care power of attorney and a living will, do not use the supplement from Appendix B. Instead, staple the Arizona living will form from Appendix D to the back of your power of attorney. If you do not make a power of attorney, use the supplement and staple it to the back of the living will form from Appendix D.

Minnesota: In the "Health Care Declaration" form, in spaces (1), (3), (5), (6) and (7) print or write "I want the attached Supplement to Directive or Declaration to Physicians and Durable Power of Attorney for Health-Care Decisions to be part of this document." In spaces (2) and (4) of the form, either write what you wish or put an X across the space. In space (8) of the form, fill in the name, address, telephone number and relationship of your agent and alternate agent.

Nebraska: In each of the three places where the state "Power of Attorney for Health Care" form has "I direct that" followed by blank lines, print or write "See my Durable Power Of Attorney For Health-Care Decisions."

Oklahoma: In the form titled "Advance Directive for Health Care," in part "I. Living Will," in the space at b. (3), write "See my Supplement to Directive or Declaration to Physicians." In part "II. My Appointment of My Health Care Proxy," in the spaces at b. (3) and c. (3), write "See my Durable Power of Attorney for Health-Care Decisions."

South Dakota: In the form titled "Living Will Declaration," initial or put dashes in each of the treatment option spaces. Then in the space after the statement "If you do not agree with any of the printed directives and want to write your own, or if you want to write directives in addition to the printed provisions, or if you want to express some of your own thoughts you can do so here," write "See my Supplement to Directive or Declaration to Physicians."

Utah: If you want to use the model durable power of attorney in Appendix A, then in the Utah form titled "SPECIAL POWER OF ATTORNEY," in the space after "Statement of my intentions," write "I do not want my agent's authority to be limited as stated above. I want my agent to have the authority provided in my Durable Power of attorney for Health Care Decisions."

West Virginia: In the form titled "Medical Power of Attorney," at the statement "SPECIAL DIRECTIVES OR LIMITATIONS ON THIS POWER: (If none, write 'none.')," draw a line through the words from "OR" through "none," so that only the words "SPECIAL DIRECTIVES" remain. Then write or print in the space, "I want my Durable Power of Attorney for Health-Care Decisions to be treated as part of this document."

In the states listed below, print or write the statement, "I want my Durable Power of Attorney for Health-Care Decisions to be treated as part of this document," as follows:

California In the "Statutory Form Durable Power of Attorney for Health Care," at 4 (a) and (b).

Colorado In the "Document Concerning the Appointment of Health Care Agent," on the lines after "Other."

Idaho In the form titled "A Durable Power of Attorney for Health Care," on the blank line in part "4. Statement of Desires, Special Provisions, and Limitations."

Kansas In the form titled "Durable Power of Attorney for Health Care Decisions General Statement of Authority Granted," on the line after "In exercising the grant of authority set forth above my agent for health care decisions shall."

Nevada In the Nevada form titled "Durable Power of Attorney for Health Care Decisions," in the space in "4. SPECIAL PROVISIONS AND LIMITATIONS," and in the space at the end of "6. STATEMENT OF DESIRES," where the form says "Other or Additional Statements of Desires."

New Hampshire In the New Hampshire form that begins with "Information Concerning the Durable Power of Attorney for Health Care," in the space in part 4.

North Dakota In the form titled "Statutory Form Durable Power of Attorney for Health Care," in the spaces in part 4. at a. and b.

Oregon In the form titled "Power of Attorney for Health Care," in the space after "I direct that my attorney-in-fact comply with the following instructions or limitations." Also initial the two options after that space, if they reflect your intentions.

Rhode Island In the form titled "Statutory Form Durable Power of Attorney for Health Care," in part "(4) STATEMENT OF DESIRES, SPECIAL PROVISIONS, AND LIMITATIONS," in the spaces after (a) and (b).

South Carolina In the form titled "Health Care Power of Attorney," in part 6 at part (4), in the space following the statement "Directive in my own words." Also in part 6, most people will want to initial option "(1) GRANT OF DISCRETION TO AGENT" or "(2) DIRECTIVE TO WITHHOLD OR WITHDRAW TREATMENT" (it is ok to initial both even though the form indicates to choose between them) and cross out option "(3) DIRECTIVE FOR MAXIMUM TREATMENT." If you do not want to limit your agent's powers, make an X across the space at part 3. E. in that form.

Texas In the Texas form that begins with "Information Concerning the Durable Power of Attorney for Health Care" in the space after "Further statement of intentions," before the signature line. Also, if you do not want to place any restrictions on your agent's authority, then after the statement "LIMITATIONS ON THE DECISION MAKING AUTHORITY OF MY AGENT ARE AS FOLLOWS," write "None."

Vermont In the document titled "Durable Power of Attorney for Health Care," in the space after "(a) STATEMENT OF DESIRES, SPECIAL PROVISIONS, AND LIMITATIONS REGARDING HEALTH CARE DECISIONS."

Virginia In the form titled "Advance Medical Directive," in the space after "F. Other statements."

Wisconsin In the form that starts with "NOTICE TO PERSON MAKING THIS DOCUMENT (HEALTH CARE POWER OF ATTORNEY)," in the space after "STATEMENT OF DESIRES, SPECIAL PROVISIONS OR LIMITATIONS."

Declaration

Declaration made this _____ day of _____ (month, year). I, _____, being of sound mind, willfully and voluntarily make known my desires that my dying shall not be artificially prolonged under the circumstances set forth below, do hereby declare:

If at any time I should have an incurable injury, disease, or illness certified to be a terminal condition by two physicians who have personally examined me, one of whom shall be my attending physician, and the physicians have determined that my death will occur whether or not life-sustaining procedures are utilized and where the application of life-sustaining procedures would serve only to artificially prolong the dying process, I direct that such procedures be withheld or withdrawn, and that I be permitted to die naturally with only the administration of medication or the performance of any medical procedure deemed necessary to provide me with comfort care.

In the absence of my ability to give directions regarding the use of such life-sustaining procedures, it is my intention that this declaration shall be honored by my family and physician(s) as the final expression of my legal right to refuse medical or surgical treatment and accept the consequences from such refusal.

I understand the full import of this declaration and I am emotionally and mentally competent to make this declaration.

Signed _____

City, County and State of Residence _____

_____

Date _____

The declarant has been personally known to me and I believe him or her to be of sound mind. I did not sign the declarant's signature above for or at the direction of the declarant. I am not related to the declarant by blood or marriage, entitled to any portion of the estate of the declarant according to the laws of intestate succession or under any will of declarant or codicil thereto, or directly financially responsible for declarant's medical care.

Witness _____

Address _____

Telephone _____

Date _____

Witness _____

Address _____

Telephone _____

Date _____

ALASKA

Declaration

If I should have an incurable or irreversible condition that will cause my death within a relatively short time, it is my desire that my life not be prolonged by administration of life-sustaining procedures.

If my condition is terminal and I am unable to participate in decisions regarding my medical treatment, I direct my attending physician to withhold or withdraw procedures that merely prolong the dying process and are not necessary to my comfort or to alleviate pain.

I [   ] do [   ] do not desire that nutrition or hydration (food and water) be provided by gastric tube or intravenously if necessary.

Signed this _____ day of _____, _____.

Signature _____

Place _____

The declarant is known to me and voluntarily signed or voluntarily directed another to sign this document in my presence.

Witness _____

Address _____

Telephone _____

Witness _____

Address _____

Telephone _____

State of _____

_____ Judicial District

The foregoing instrument was acknowledged before me this (date) by (name of person who acknowledged).

_____
Signature of Person Taking
Acknowledgement

_____
Title or Rank

_____
Serial Number, if any

THIS DECLARATION MUST BE EITHER WITNESSED BY TWO PERSONS OR ACKNOWLEDGED BY A PERSON QUALIFIED TO TAKE ACKNOWLEDGEMENTS UNDER AS 09.63.010.

Living Will

(SOME GENERAL STATEMENTS CONCERNING YOUR HEALTH CARE OPTIONS ARE OUTLINED BELOW. IF YOU AGREE WITH ONE OF THE STATEMENTS, YOU SHOULD INITIAL THAT STATEMENT. READ ALL OF THESE STATEMENTS CAREFULLY BEFORE YOU INITIAL YOUR SELECTION. YOU CAN ALSO WRITE YOUR OWN STATEMENT CONCERNING LIFE-SUSTAINING TREATMENT AND OTHER MATTERS RELATING TO YOUR HEALTH CARE. YOU MAY INITIAL ANY COMBINATION OF PARAGRAPHS 1, 2 AND 3, BUT IF YOU INITIAL PARAGRAPH 4 THE OTHERS SHOULD *NOT* BE INITIALED.)

_____ 1. IF I HAVE A TERMINAL CONDITION I DO NOT WANT MY LIFE TO BE PROLONGED, AND I DO NOT WANT LIFE-SUSTAINING TREATMENT, BEYOND COMFORT CARE, THAT WOULD SERVE ONLY TO ARTIFICIALLY DELAY THE MOMENT OF MY DEATH.

_____ 2. IF I AM IN A TERMINAL CONDITION OR AN IRREVERSIBLE COMA OR A PERSISTENT VEGETATIVE STATE THAT MY DOCTORS REASONABLY FEEL TO BE IRREVERSIBLE OR INCURABLE, I DO WANT THE MEDICAL TREATMENT NECESSARY TO PROVIDE CARE THAT WOULD KEEP ME COMFORTABLE, BUT I DO NOT WANT THE FOLLOWING:

  _____ (a) CARDIOPULMONARY RESUSCITATION, FOR EXAMPLE, THE USE OF DRUGS, ELECTRIC SHOCK AND ARTIFICIAL BREATHING.

  _____ (b) ARTIFICIALLY ADMINISTERED FOOD AND FLUIDS.

  _____ (c) TO BE TAKEN TO A HOSPITAL IF AT ALL AVOIDABLE.

_____ 3. NOTWITHSTANDING MY OTHER DIRECTIONS, IF I AM KNOWN TO BE PREGNANT, I DO NOT WANT LIFE-SUSTAINING TREATMENT WITHHELD OR WITHDRAWN IF IT IS POSSIBLE THAT THE EMBRYO/FETUS WILL DEVELOP TO THE POINT OF LIVE BIRTH WITH THE CONTINUED APPLICATION OF LIFE-SUSTAINING TREATMENT.

_____ 4. NOTWITHSTANDING MY OTHER DIRECTIONS I *DO* WANT THE USE OF ALL MEDICAL CARE NECESSARY TO TREAT MY CONDITION UNTIL MY DOCTORS REASONABLY CONCLUDE THAT MY CONDITION IS TERMINAL OR IS IRREVERSIBLE AND INCURABLE OR I AM IN A PERSISTENT VEGETATIVE STATE.

_____ 5. I WANT MY LIFE TO BE PROLONGED TO THE GREATEST EXTENT POSSIBLE.

_____   _____

Signature   Date

Witness Name _____

Address _____

Telephone _____

Witness Name _____
(optional)

Address _____

Telephone _____

Arizona

or

Notarization. Signed, acknowledged, and sworn before me this ———————————————— day of
————————————, 199——. Notary Public for the State of Arizona, county of ————————————————,
residing at ——————————————.

————————————————————————
Notary. My commission expires ——————————————.

Declaration

If I should have an incurable or irreversible condition that will cause my death within a relatively short time, or, if I should become permanently unconscious, and I am no longer able to make decisions regarding my medical treatment, I direct my attending physician, pursuant to the Arkansas Rights of the Terminally Ill or Permanently Unconscious Act, to withhold or withdraw treatment that only prolongs the process of dying and is not necessary to my comfort or to alleviate pain and to follow the instructions of _____ whom I appoint as my Health Care Proxy to decide whether life-sustaining treatment should be withheld or withdrawn.

Signed this _____ day of _____, _____

Signature _____

Address _____

The declarant voluntarily signed this writing in my presence.

Witness _____

Address _____

Telephone _____

Witness _____

Address _____

Telephone _____

Statutory Form Durable Power of Attorney for Health Care (California Civil Code Section 2500)

WARNING TO PERSON EXECUTING THIS DOCUMENT

THIS IS AN IMPORTANT LEGAL DOCUMENT WHICH IS AUTHORIZED BY THE KEENE HEALTH CARE AGENT ACT. BEFORE EXECUTING THIS DOCUMENT, YOU SHOULD KNOW THESE IMPORTANT FACTS:

THIS DOCUMENT GIVES THE PERSON YOU DESIGNATE AS YOUR AGENT (THE ATTORNEY IN FACT) THE POWER TO MAKE HEALTH CARE DECISIONS FOR YOU. YOUR AGENT MUST ACT CONSISTENTLY WITH YOUR DESIRES AS STATED IN THIS DOCUMENT OR OTHERWISE MADE KNOWN.

EXCEPT AS YOU OTHERWISE SPECIFY IN THIS DOCUMENT, THIS DOCUMENT GIVES YOUR AGENT THE POWER TO CONSENT TO YOUR DOCTOR NOT GIVING TREATMENT OR STOPPING TREATMENT NECESSARY TO KEEP YOU ALIVE.

NOTWITHSTANDING THIS DOCUMENT, YOU HAVE THE RIGHT TO MAKE MEDICAL AND OTHER HEALTH CARE DECISIONS FOR YOURSELF SO LONG AS YOU CAN GIVE INFORMED CONSENT WITH RESPECT TO THE PARTICULAR DECISION. IN ADDITION, NO TREATMENT MAY BE GIVEN TO YOU OVER YOUR OBJECTION AT THE TIME, AND HEALTH CARE NECESSARY TO KEEP YOU ALIVE MAY NOT BE STOPPED OR WITHHELD IF YOU OBJECT AT THE TIME.

THIS DOCUMENT GIVES YOUR AGENT AUTHORITY TO CONSENT, TO REFUSE TO CONSENT, OR TO WITHDRAW CONSENT TO ANY CARE, TREATMENT, SERVICE, OR PROCEDURE TO MAINTAIN, DIAGNOSE, OR TREAT A PHYSICAL OR MENTAL CONDITION. THIS POWER IS SUBJECT TO ANY STATEMENT OF YOUR DESIRES AND ANY LIMITATIONS THAT YOU INCLUDE IN THIS DOCUMENT. YOU MAY STATE IN THIS DOCUMENT ANY TYPES OF TREATMENT THAT YOU DO NOT DESIRE. IN ADDITION, A COURT CAN TAKE AWAY THE POWER OF YOUR AGENT TO MAKE HEALTH CARE DECISIONS FOR YOU IF YOUR AGENT (1) AUTHORIZES ANYTHING THAT IS ILLEGAL, (2) ACTS CONTRARY TO YOUR KNOWN DESIRES, OR (3) WHERE YOUR DESIRES ARE NOT KNOWN, DOES ANYTHING THAT IS CLEARLY CONTRARY TO YOUR BEST INTERESTS.

THE POWERS GIVEN BY THIS DOCUMENT WILL EXIST FOR AN INDEFINITE PERIOD OF TIME UNLESS YOU LIMIT THEIR DURATION IN THIS DOCUMENT.

YOU HAVE THE RIGHT TO REVOKE THE AUTHORITY OF YOUR AGENT BY NOTIFYING YOUR AGENT OR YOUR TREATING DOCTOR, HOSPITAL, OR OTHER HEALTH CARE PROVIDER ORALLY OR IN WRITING OF THE REVOCATION.

YOUR AGENT HAS THE RIGHT TO EXAMINE YOUR MEDICAL RECORDS AND TO CONSENT TO THEIR DISCLOSURE UNLESS YOU LIMIT THIS RIGHT IN THIS DOCUMENT.

UNLESS YOU OTHERWISE SPECIFY IN THIS DOCUMENT, THIS DOCUMENT GIVES YOUR AGENT THE POWER AFTER YOU DIE TO (1) AUTHORIZE AN AUTOPSY, (2) DONATE YOUR BODY OR

PARTS THEREOF FOR TRANSPLANT OR THERAPEUTIC OR EDUCATIONAL OR SCIENTIFIC PURPOSES, AND (3) DIRECT THE DISPOSITION OF YOUR REMAINS.

THIS DOCUMENT REVOKES ANY PRIOR DURABLE POWER OF ATTORNEY FOR HEALTH CARE.

YOU SHOULD CAREFULLY READ AND FOLLOW THE WITNESSING PROCEDURE DESCRIBED AT THE END OF THIS FORM. THIS DOCUMENT WILL NOT BE VALID UNLESS YOU COMPLY WITH THE WITNESSING PROCEDURE.

IF THERE IS ANYTHING IN THIS DOCUMENT THAT YOU DO NOT UNDERSTAND, YOU SHOULD ASK A LAWYER TO EXPLAIN IT TO YOU.

YOUR AGENT MAY NEED THIS DOCUMENT IMMEDIATELY IN CASE OF AN EMERGENCY THAT REQUIRES A DECISION CONCERNING YOUR HEALTH CARE. EITHER KEEP THIS DOCUMENT WHERE IT IS IMMEDIATELY AVAILABLE TO YOUR AGENT AND ALTERNATE AGENTS OR GIVE EACH OF THEM AN EXECUTED COPY OF THIS DOCUMENT. YOU MAY ALSO WANT TO GIVE YOUR DOCTOR AN EXECUTED COPY OF THIS DOCUMENT.

DO NOT USE THIS FORM IF YOU ARE A CONSERVATEE UNDER THE LANTERMAN-PETRIS-SHORT ACT AND YOU WANT TO APPOINT YOUR CONSERVATOR AS YOUR AGENT. YOU CAN DO THAT ONLY IF THE APPOINTMENT DOCUMENT INCLUDES A CERTIFICATE OF YOUR ATTORNEY.

1. DESIGNATION OF HEALTH CARE AGENT. I, _____

_____

(Insert your name and address)

do hereby designate and appoint _____

_____

(Insert name, address, and telephone number of one individual only as your agent to make health care decisions for you. None of the following may be designated as your agent: (1) your treating health care provider, (2) a nonrelative employee of your treating health care provider, (3) an operator of a community care facility, (4) a nonrelative employee of an operator of a community care facility, (5) an operator of a residential care facility for the elderly, or (6) a nonrelative employee of an operator of a residential care facility for the elderly.) as my attorney in fact (agent) to make health care decisions for me as authorized in this document. For the purposes of this document, "health care decision" means consent, refusal of consent, or withdrawal of consent to any care, treatment, service, or procedure to maintain, diagnose, or treat an individual's physical or mental condition.

2. CREATION OF DURABLE POWER OF ATTORNEY FOR HEALTH CARE. By this document I intend to create a durable power of attorney for health care under Sections 2430 to 2443, inclusive, of the California Civil Code. This power of attorney is authorized by the Keene Health Care Agent Act and shall be construed in accordance with the provisions of Sections 2500 to 2506, inclusive, of the California Civil Code. This power of attorney shall not be affected by my subsequent incapacity.

3. GENERAL STATEMENT OF AUTHORITY GRANTED. Subject to any limitations in this document, I hereby grant to my agent full power and authority to make health care decisions for me to the same extent that I could make such decisions for myself if I had the capacity to do so. In exercising this authority, my agent shall make health care decisions that are consistent with my desires as stated in this document or otherwise made known to my agent, including, but not limited to, my desires concerning obtaining or refusing or withdrawing life-prolonging care, treatment services, and procedures.

(If you want to limit the authority of your agent to make health care decisions for you, you can state the limitations in paragraph 4 ("Statement of Desires, Special Provisions, and Limitations") below. You can indicate your desires by including a statement of your desires in the same paragraph.)

4. STATEMENT OF DESIRES, SPECIAL PROVISIONS, AND LIMITATIONS. (Your agent must make health care decisions that are consistent with your known desires. You can, but are not required to, state

your desires in the space provided below. You should consider whether you want to include a statement of your desires concerning life-prolonging care, treatment, services, and procedures. You can also include a statement of your desires concerning other matters relating to your health care. You can also make your desires known to your agent by discussing your desires with your agent or by some other means. If there are any types of treatment that you do not want to be used, you should state them in the space below. If you want to limit in any other way the authority given your agent by this document, you should state the limits in the space below. If you do not state any limits, your agent will have broad powers to make health care decisions for you, except to the extent that there are limits provided by law.)

In exercising the authority under this durable power of attorney for health care, my agent shall act consistently with my desires as stated below and is subject to the special provisions and limitations stated below:

(a) Statement of desires concerning life-prolonging care, treatment, services, and procedures:

_____

_____

_____

_____

_____

_____

_____

_____

(b) Additional statement of desires, special provisions, and limitations: _____

_____

_____

_____

_____

_____

_____

_____

_____

_____

(You may attach additional pages if you need more space to complete your statement. If you attach additional pages, you must date and sign EACH of the additional pages at the same time you date and sign this document.)

5. INSPECTION AND DISCLOSURE OF INFORMATION RELATING TO MY PHYSICAL OR MENTAL HEALTH. Subject to any limitations in this document, my agent has the power and authority to do all of the following.

(a) Request, review, and receive any information, verbal or written, regarding my physical or mental health, including, but not limited to, medical and hospital records.

(b) Execute on my behalf any releases or other documents that may be required in order to obtain this information.

(c) Consent to the disclosure of this information.

(If you want to limit the authority of your agent to receive and disclose information relating to your health, you must state the limitations in paragraph 4 ("Statement of Desires, Special Provisions, and Limitations") above.)

6. SIGNING DOCUMENTS, WAIVERS, AND RELEASES. When necessary to implement the health care decisions that my agent is authorized by this document to make, my agent has the power and authority to execute on my behalf all of the following:

(a) Documents titled or purporting to be a "Refusal to Permit Treatment" and "Leaving Hospital Against Medical Advice."

(b) Any necessary waiver or release from liability required by a hospital or physician.

7. AUTOPSY; ANATOMICAL GIFTS; DISPOSITION OF REMAINS. Subject to any limitations in this document, my agent has the power and authority to do all of the following:

(a) Authorize an autopsy under Section 7113 of the Health and Safety Code.

(b) Make a disposition of a part or parts of my body under the Uniform Anatomical Gift Act (Chapter 3.5 (commencing with Section 7150) of Part 1 of Division 7 of the Health and Safety Code).

(c) Direct the disposition of my remains under Section 7100 of the Health and Safety Code.

(If you want to limit the authority of your agent to consent to an autopsy, make an anatomical gift, or direct the disposition of your remains, you must state the limitations in paragraph 4 ("Statement of Desires, Special Provisions, and Limitations") above.)

8. DURATION.

(Unless you specify otherwise in the space below, this power of attorney will exist for an indefinite period of time.)

This durable power of attorney for health care expires on _____

_____

(Fill in this space ONLY if you want to limit the duration of this power of attorney.)

9. DESIGNATION OF ALTERNATE AGENTS.

(You are not required to designate any alternate agents but you may do so. Any alternate agent you designate will be able to make the same health care decisions as the agent you designated in paragraph 1, above, in the event that agent is unable or ineligible to act as your agent. If the agent you designated is your spouse, he or she becomes ineligible to act as your agent if your marriage is dissolved.)

If the person designated as my agent in paragraph 1 is not available or becomes ineligible to act as my agent to make a health care decision for me or loses the mental capacity to make health care decisions for me, or if I revoke that person's appointment or authority to act as my agent to make health care decisions for me, then I designate and appoint the following persons to serve as my agent to make health care decisions for me as authorized in this document, such persons to serve in the order listed below:

A. First Alternate Agent _____

_____

(Insert name, address, and telephone number of first alternate agent)

B. Second Alternate Agent _____

_____

(Insert name, address, and telephone number of second alternate agent)

10. NOMINATION OF CONSERVATOR OF PERSON.

(A conservator of the person may be appointed for you if a court decides that one should be appointed. The conservator is responsible for your physical care, which under some circumstances includes making health care decisions for you. You are not required to nominate a conservator but you may do so. The court will appoint the person you nominate unless that would be contrary to your best interests. You may, but are not required to, nominate as your conservator the same person you named in paragraph 1 as your health care agent. You can nominate an individual as your conservator by completing the space below.)

If a conservator of the person is to be appointed for me, I nominate the following individual to serve as conservator of the person _____

_____

(Insert name and address of person nominated as conservator of the person)

11. PRIOR DESIGNATIONS REVOKED. I revoke any prior durable power of attorney for health care.

DATE AND SIGNATURE OF PRINCIPAL
(YOU MUST DATE AND SIGN THIS POWER OF ATTORNEY)
I sign my name to this Statutory Form Durable Power of Attorney for Health Care on

Date _____

City _____

State _____

You sign here _____

(THIS POWER OF ATTORNEY WILL NOT BE VALID UNLESS IT IS SIGNED BY TWO QUALIFIED WITNESSES WHO ARE PRESENT WHEN YOU SIGN OR ACKNOWLEDGE YOUR SIGNATURE. IF YOU HAVE ATTACHED ANY ADDITIONAL PAGES TO THIS FORM, YOU MUST DATE AND SIGN EACH OF THE ADDITIONAL PAGES AT THE SAME TIME YOU DATE AND SIGN THIS POWER OF ATTORNEY.)

STATEMENT OF WITNESSES

(This document must be witnessed by two qualified adult witnesses. None of the following may be used as witness: (1) a person you designate as your agent or alternate agent, (2) a health care provider, (3) an employee of a health care provider, (4) the operator of a community care facility, (5) an employee of an operator of a community care facility, (6) the operator of a residential care facility for the elderly, or (7) an employee of an operator of a residential care facility for the elderly. At least one of the witnesses must make the additional declaration set out following the place where the witnesses sign.)

(READ CAREFULLY BEFORE SIGNING. You can sign as a witness only if you personally know the principal or the identity of the principal is proved to you by convincing evidence.)

(To have convincing evidence of the identity of the principal, you must be presented with and reasonably rely on any one or more of the following:

(1) An identification card or driver's license issued by the California Department of Motor Vehicles that is current or has been issued within five years.

(2) A passport issued by the Department of State of the United States that is current or has been issued within five years.

(3) Any of the following documents if the document is current or has been issued within five years and contains a photograph and description of the person named on it, is signed by the person, and bears a serial or other identifying number.

(a) A passport issued by a foreign government that has been stamped by the United States Immigration and Naturalization Service.

(b) A driver's license issued by a state other than California or by a Canadian or Mexican public agency authorized to issue drivers' licenses.

(c) An identification card issued by a state other than California.

(d) An identification card issued by any branch of the armed forces of the United States.

(4) If the principal is a patient in a skilled nursing facility, a witness who is a patient advocate or ombudsman may rely upon the representations of the administrator or staff of the skilled nursing facility, or of family members, as convincing evidence of the identity of the principal if the patient advocate or ombudsman believes that the representations provide a reasonable basis for determining the identity of the principal.)

(Other kinds of proof of identity are not allowed.)

I declare under penalty of perjury under the laws of California that the person who signed or acknowledged this document is personally known to me (or proved to me on the basis of convincing evidence) to be the principal, that the principal signed or acknowledged this durable power of attorney in my presence, that the principal appears to be of sound mind and under no duress, fraud, or undue influence, that I am not the person appointed as attorney in fact by this document, and that I am not a health care provider, an employee of a health care provider, the operator of a community care facility, an employee of an operator of a community care facility, the operator of a residential care facility for the elderly, nor an employee of an operator of a residential care facility for the elderly.

Signature: _____

Print Name: _____

Date: _____

Residence Address: _____

_____

Telephone: _____

Signature: _____

Print Name: _____

Date: _____

Residence Address: _____

_____

Telephone: _____

(AT LEAST ONE OF THE ABOVE WITNESSES MUST ALSO SIGN THE FOLLOWING DECLARATION.)

I further declare under penalty of perjury under the laws of California that I am not related to the principal by blood, marriage, or adoption, and, to the best of my knowledge, I am not entitled to any part of the estate of the principal upon the death of the principal under a will now existing or by operation of law.

Signature: _____

Signature: _____

STATEMENT OF PATIENT ADVOCATE OR OMBUDSMAN

(If you are a patient in a skilled nursing facility, one of the witnesses must be a patient advocate or ombudsman. The following statement is required only if you are a patient in a skilled nursing facility—a health care facility that provides the following basic services: skilled nursing care and supportive care to patients whose primary need is for availability of skilled nursing care on an extended basis. The patient advocate or ombudsman must sign both parts of the "Statement of Witnesses" above AND must also sign the following statement.)

I further declare under penalty of perjury under the laws of California that I am a patient advocate or ombudsman as designated by the State Department of Aging and that I am serving as a witness as required by subdivision (f) of Section 2432 of the Civil Code.

Signature: _____

Declaration

If I should have an incurable and irreversible condition that has been diagnosed by two physicians and that will result in my death within a relatively short time without the administration of life-sustaining treatment or has produced an irreversible coma or persistent vegetative state, and I am no longer able to make decisions regarding my medical treatment, I direct my attending physician, pursuant to the Natural Death Act of California, to withhold or withdraw treatment, including artificially administered nutrition and hydration, that only prolongs the process of dying or the irreversible coma or persistent vegetative state and is not necessary for my comfort or to alleviate pain.

If I have been diagnosed as pregnant, and that diagnosis is known to my physician, this declaration shall have no force or effect during my pregnancy.

Signed this _____ day of _____, 199___.

Signature _____

Address _____

The declarant voluntarily signed this writing in my presence. I am not a health care provider, an employee of a health care provider, the operator of a community care facility, an employee of an operator of a community care facility, the operator of a residential care facility for the elderly, or an employee of an operator of a residential care facility for the elderly.

Witness _____

Address _____

Telephone _____

The declarant voluntarily signed this writing in my presence. I am not entitled to any portion of the estate of the declarant upon his or her death under any will or codicil thereto of the declarant now existing or by operation of law. I am not a health care provider, an employee of a health care provider, the operator of a community care facility, an employee of an operator of a community care facility, the operator of a residential care facility for the elderly, or an employee of an operator of a residential care facility for the elderly.

Witness _____

Address _____

Telephone _____

Declaration as to Medical or Surgical Treatment

I, _____, being of sound mind and at least eighteen years of age, direct that my life shall not be artificially prolonged under the circumstances set forth below and hereby declare that:

1. If at any time my attending physician and one other qualified physician certify in writing that:

a. I have an injury, disease, or illness which is not curable or reversible and which, in their judgment, is a terminal condition, and

b. For a period of seven consecutive days or more, I have been unconscious, comatose, or otherwise incompetent so as to be unable to make or communicate responsible decisions concerning my person, then

I direct that, in accordance with Colorado law, life-sustaining procedures shall be withdrawn and withheld pursuant to the terms of this declaration, it being understood that life-sustaining procedures shall not include any medical procedure or intervention for nourishment considered necessary by the attending physician to provide comfort or alleviate pain. However, I may specifically direct, in accordance with Colorado law, that artificial nourishment be withdrawn or withheld pursuant to the terms of this declaration.

2. In the event that the only procedure I am being provided is artificial nourishment, I direct that one of the following actions be taken (initial one):

(_____) a. Artificial nourishment shall not be continued when it is the only procedure being provided; or

(_____) b. Artificial nourishment shall be continued for _____ days when it is the only procedure being provided; or

(_____) c. Artificial nourishment shall be continued when it is the only procedure being provided.

3. I execute this declaration, as my free and voluntary act, this _____ day of _____, 19___.

By _____
Declarant

The foregoing instrument was signed and declared by _____ to be his declaration, in the presence of us, who, in his presence, in the presence of each other, and at his request, have signed our names below as witnesses, and we declare that, at the time of the execution of this instrument, the declarant, according to our best knowledge and belief, was of sound mind and under no constraint or undue influence.

Dated at _____, Colorado, this _____ day of _____, 19___.

_____
Witness (Name, Address, and Telephone)

_____
Witness (Name, Address, and Telephone)

Colorado

STATE OF COLORADO   )
) ss.

County of _____)

     SUBSCRIBED and sworn to before me by _____, the declarant, and _____ and _____, witnesses, as the voluntary act and deed of the declarant this _____ day of _____, 19__.

My commission expires:

_____
                                                   Notary Public

Document Concerning the Appointment of Health Care Agent

I appoint _____ (name) to be my health care agent. If my attending physician determines that I am unable to understand and appreciate the nature and consequences of health care decisions and to reach and communicate an informed decision regarding treatment, my health care agent is authorized to:

    (1) Convey to my physician my wishes concerning the withholding or removal of life support systems.

    (2) Take whatever actions are necessary to ensure that my wishes are given effect.

Other: _____

_____

    If this person is unwilling or unable to serve as my health care agent, I appoint _____ _____ (name) to be my alternative health care agent.

    This request is made, after careful reflection, while I am of sound mind.

Signature _____

Date _____

    This document was signed in our presence, by the above-named _____ (name) who appeared to be eighteen years of age or older, of sound mind and able to understand the nature and consequences of health care decisions at the time the document was signed.

Witness _____

Date _____

Address _____

Telephone _____

Witness _____

Date _____

Address _____

Telephone _____

CONNECTICUT _____

Document Concerning Withholding or Withdrawal of Life Support Systems (Living Will)

If the time comes when I am incapacitated to the point when I can no longer actively take part in decisions for my own life, and am unable to direct my physician as to my own medical care, I wish this statement to stand as a testament of my wishes.

I, _____ (name), request that, if my condition is deemed terminal or if I am determined to be permanently unconscious, I be allowed to die and not be kept alive through life support systems. By terminal condition, I mean that I have an incurable or irreversible medical condition which, without the administration of life support systems, will, in the opinion of my attending physician, result in death within a relatively short time. By permanently unconscious I mean that I am in a permanent coma or persistent vegetative state which is an irreversible condition in which I am at no time aware of myself or the environment and show no behavioral response to the environment. The life support systems which I do not want include, but are not limited to:

Artificial respiration

Cardiopulmonary resuscitation

Artificial means of providing nutrition and hydration

(Cross out and initial life support systems you want administered)

I do not intend any direct taking of my life, but only that my dying not be unreasonably prolonged. Other specific requests:

This request is made, after careful reflection, while I am of sound mind.

(signature) _____

(date) _____

This document was signed in our presence, by the above-named _____ (name) who appeared to be eighteen years of age or older, of sound mind and able to understand the nature and consequences of health care decisions at the time the document was signed.

(Witness) _____

(Address) _____

(Telephone) _____

(Witness) _____

(Address) _____

(Telephone) _____

DISTRICT OF COLUMBIA

Declaration

Declaration made this _____ day of _____ (month, year).

    I, _____, being of sound mind, willfully and voluntarily make known my desires that my dying shall not be artificially prolonged under the circumstances set forth below, do declare:

    If at any time I should have an incurable injury, disease, or illness certified to be a terminal condition by 2 physicians who have personally examined me, one of whom shall be my attending physician, and the physicians have determined that my death will occur whether or not life-sustaining procedures are utilized and where the application of life-sustaining procedures would serve only to artificially prolong the dying process, I direct that such procedures be withheld or withdrawn, and that I be permitted to die naturally with only the administration of medication or the performance of any medical procedure deemed necessary to provide me with comfort care or to alleviate pain.

    In the absence of my ability to give directions regarding the use of such life-sustaining procedures, it is my intention that this declaration shall be honored by my family and physician(s) as the final expression of my legal right to refuse medical or surgical treatment and accept the consequences from such refusal.

    I understand the full import of this declaration and I am emotionally and mentally competent to make this declaration.

Signed _____

Address _____

    I believe the declarant to be of sound mind. I did not sign the declarant's signature above for or at the direction of the declarant. I am least 18 years of age and am not related to the declarant by blood or marriage, entitled to any portion of the estate of the declarant according to the laws of intestate succession of the District of Columbia or under any will of the declarant or codicil thereto, or directly financially responsible for declarant's medical care. I am not the declarant's attending physician, an employee of the attending physician, or an employee of the health facility in which the declarant is a patient.

Witness (name) _____

(address) _____

(telephone) _____

Witness (name) _____

(address) _____

(telephone) _____

Living Will

Declaration made this _____ day of _____ 19_____. I
_____ willfully and voluntarily make known my desire that my dying not be
artificially prolonged under the circumstances set forth below, and I do hereby declare:

If at any time I have a terminal condition and if my attending or treating physician and another
consulting physician have determined that there is no medical probability of my recovery from such
condition. I direct that life-prolonging procedures be withheld or withdrawn when the application of such
procedures would serve only to prolong artificially the process of dying, and that I be permitted to die
naturally with only the administration of medication or the performance of any medical procedure deemed
necessary to provide me with comfort care or to alleviate pain.

It is my intention that this declaration be honored by my family and physician as the final expression of
my legal right to refuse medical or surgical treatment and to accept the consequences for such refusal.

In the event that I have been determined to be unable to provide express and informed consent regarding the withholding, withdrawal, or continuation of life-prolonging procedures, I wish to designate, as my
surrogate to carry out the provisions of this declaration:

Name: _____

Address: _____

Phone: _____

I understand the full import of this declaration, and I am emotionally and mentally competent to make
this declaration.

Additional Instructions (optional):

_____

_____

_____

_____   _____

Signature   Date

Witnesses:

Name _____   Name _____

Telephone _____   Telephone _____

Address _____   Address _____

_____   _____

Living Will

Living will made this _____ day of _____ (month, year).

I, _____, being of sound mind, willfully and voluntarily make known my desire that my life shall not be prolonged under the circumstances set forth below and do declare:

1. If at any time I should (check each option desired):

(_____) have a terminal condition,

(_____) become in a coma with no reasonable expectation of regaining consciousness, or

(_____) become in a persistent vegetative state with no reasonable expectation of regaining significant cognitive function,

as defined in and established in accordance with the procedures set forth in paragraphs (2), (9), and (10) of Code Section 31-32-2 of the Official Code of Georgia Annotated, I direct that the application of life-sustaining procedures to my body (check the option desired):

(_____) including nourishment and hydration,

(_____) including hydration but not nourishment, or

(_____) excluding nourishment and hydration,

be withheld or withdrawn and that I be permitted to die;

2. In the absence of my ability to give directions regarding the use of such life-sustaining procedures, it is my intention that this living will shall be honored by my family and physician(s) as the final expression of my legal right to refuse medical or surgical treatment and accept the consequences from such refusal;

3. I understand that I may revoke this living will at any time;

4. I understand the full import of this living will, and I am at least 18 years of age and am emotionally and mentally competent to make this living will; and

5. If I am a female and I have been diagnosed as pregnant, this living will shall have no force and effect unless the fetus is not viable and I indicate by initialing after this sentence that I want this living will to be carried out. _____ (Initial)

Signed _____

(City) _____

(County) _____

(State of Residence) _____

I hereby witness this living will and attest that:

(1) The declarant is personally known to me and I believe the declarant to be at least 18 years of age and of sound mind;

(2) I am at least 18 years of age;

(3) To the best of my knowledge, at the time of the execution of this living will, I:

(A) Am not related to the declarant by blood or marriage;

(B) Would not be entitled to any portion of the declarant's estate by any will or by operation of law under the rules of descent and distribution of this state;

Georgia

(C) Am not the attending physician of declarant or an employee of the attending physician or an employee of the hospital or skilled nursing facility in which declarant is a patient;

(D) Am not directly financially responsible for the declarant's medical care; and

(E) Have no present claim against any portion of the estate of the declarant;

(4) Declarant has signed this document in my presence as above-instructed, on the date above first shown.

Witness _____

Address _____

Telephone _____

Witness _____

Address _____

Telephone _____

Additional witness required when living will is signed in a hospital or skilled nursing facility.

I hereby witness this living will and attest that I believe the declarant to be of sound mind and to have made this living will willingly and voluntarily.

Witness: _____

Medical director of skilled nursing facility or staff physician not participating in care of the patient or chief of the hospital medical staff or staff physician or hospital designee not participating in care of the patient.

Declaration

A. Statement of Declarant

Declaration made this _____ day of _____ (month, year). I, _____, being of sound mind, and understanding that I have the right to request that my life be prolonged to the greatest extent possible, wilfully and voluntarily make known my desire that my dying shall not be artificially prolonged under the circumstances set forth below, and do hereby declare:

My instructions shall prevail even if they create a conflict with the desires of my relatives, hospital policies, or the principles of those providing my care.

If I should develop a terminal condition or a permanent loss of the ability to communicate concerning medical treatment decisions, with no reasonable chance of regaining this ability, I do not want to have my life prolonged. I would not want to be subjected to surgery or resuscitation. Nor would I then wish to have life sustaining medicine or procedures. Instead, I request care, including medicine and procedures, for the purpose of providing comfort and pain relief.

CHECKLIST

I have also considered whether I want tube feeding to be provided and have selected one of the following provisions by putting a mark in the space provided:

(_____) I do NOT want my life prolonged by tube or other artificial feeding or provision of fluids by a tube if my condition is as stated above.

(_____) I DO want my life prolonged by tube or other artificial feeding and provision of fluids by a tube if my condition is as stated above.

If neither provision is selected or if both are selected, it shall be presumed that tube or other artificial feeding or provision of fluids by a tube are requested to prolong the declarant's life.

This declaration shall control in all circumstances.

I understand the full import of this declaration and I am emotionally and mentally competent to make this decision.

Signed _____

Address _____

B. Statement of Witnesses

I am at least 18 years of age and

—not related to the declarant by blood, marriage, or adoption; and

—not currently the attending physician, an employee of the attending physician, or an employee of the [medical] health care facility in which the declarant is a patient.

The declarant is personally known to me and I believe the declarant to be of sound mind.

Witness _____   Witness _____

Address _____   Address _____

Telephone _____   Telephone _____

Hawaii

C. Notarization

　　Subscribed, sworn to and acknowledged before me by _____, the declarant, and subscribed and sworn to before me by _____ and _____, witnesses, this _____ day of _____, 19_____.

　　　　　　　　　　　　(SEAL)　　Signed _____

　　　　　　　　　　　　(Official capacity of officer) _____

A Living Will
A Directive to Withhold or to Provide Treatment

To my family, my relatives, my friends, my physicians, my employers, and all others whom it may concern:

Directive made this _____ day of _____ 19_____. I, _____ (name), being of sound mind, willfully, and voluntarily make known my desire that my life shall not be prolonged artificially under the circumstances set forth below, do hereby declare:

1. If at any time I should have an incurable injury, disease, illness or condition certified to be terminal by two medical doctors who have examined me, and where the application of life-sustaining procedures of any kind would serve only to prolong artificially the moment of my death, and where a medical doctor determines that my death is imminent, whether or not life-sustaining procedures are utilized, or I have been diagnosed as being in a persistent vegetative state, I direct that the following marked expression of my intent be followed and that I be permitted to die naturally, and that I receive any medical treatment or care that may be required to keep me free of pain or distress.

"Check One Box"

☐ If at any time I should become unable to communicate my instructions, then I direct that all medical treatment, care, and nutrition and hydration necessary to restore my health, sustain my life, and to abolish or alleviate pain or distress be provided to me. Nutrition and hydration shall not be withheld or withdrawn from me if I would die from malnutrition or dehydration rather than from my injury, disease, illness or condition.

☐ If at any time I should become unable to communicate my instructions and where the application of artificial life-sustaining procedures shall serve only to prolong artificially the moment of death, I direct such procedures be withheld or withdrawn except for withdrawal of the administration of nutrition and hydration.

☐ If at any time I should become unable to communicate my instructions and where the application of artificial life-sustaining procedures shall serve only to prolong artificially the moment of death, I direct such procedures be withheld or withdrawn including withdrawal of the administration of nutrition and hydration.

2. In the absence of my ability to give directions regarding the use of life-sustaining procedures, I hereby appoint _____ (name) currently residing at _____, as my attorney-in-fact/proxy for the making of decisions relating to my health care in my place; and it is my intention that this appointment shall be honored by him/her, by my family, relatives, friends, physicians and lawyer as the final expression of my legal right to refuse medical or surgical treatment; and I accept the consequences of such a decision. I have duly executed a Durable Power of Attorney for health care decisions on this date.

3. In the absence of my ability to give further directions regarding my treatment, including life-sustaining procedures, it is my intention that this directive shall be honored by my family and physicians as

the final expression of my legal right to refuse or accept medical and surgical treatment, and I accept the consequences of such refusal.

4. If I have been diagnosed as pregnant and that diagnosis is known to any interested person, this directive shall have no force during the course of my pregnancy.

5. I understand the full importance of this directive and am emotionally and mentally competent to make this directive. No participant in the making of this directive or in its being carried into effect, whether it be a medical doctor, my spouse, a relative, friend or any other person shall be held responsible in any way, legally, professionally or socially, for complying with my directions.

Signed _____

City, county and state of residence _____

The declarant has been known to me personally and I believe him/her to be of sound mind.

Witness _____

Address _____

Telephone _____

Witness _____

Address _____

Telephone _____

Declaration

This declaration is made this _____ day of _____ (month, year). I, _____, being of sound mind, willfully and voluntarily make known my desires that my moment of death shall not be artificially postponed.

If at any time I should have an incurable and irreversible injury, disease, or illness judged to be a terminal condition by my attending physician who has personally examined me and has determined that my death is imminent except for death delaying procedures, I direct that such procedures which would only prolong the dying process be withheld or withdrawn, and that I be permitted to die naturally with only the administration of medication, sustenance, or the performance of any medical procedure deemed necessary by my attending physician to provide me with comfort care.

In the absence of my ability to give directions regarding the use of such death delaying procedures, it is my intention that this declaration shall be honored by my family and physician as the final expression of my legal right to refuse medical or surgical treatment and accept the consequences from such refusal.

Signed _____

City, County and State of Residence _____

The declarant is personally known to me and I believe him or her to be of sound mind. I saw the declarant sign the declaration in my presence (or the declarant acknowledged in my presence that he or she had signed the declaration) and I signed the declaration as a witness in the presence of the declarant. I did not sign the declarant's signature above for or at the direction of the declarant. At the date of this instrument, I am not entitled to any portion of the estate of the declarant according to the laws of intestate succession or, to the best of my knowledge and belief, under any will of declarant or other instrument taking effect at declarant's death, or directly financially responsible for declarant's medical care.

Witness (name) _____

(address) _____

(telephone) _____

Witness (name) _____

(address) _____

(telephone) _____

INDIANA

Addendum to Health Care Durable Power Of Attorney

I authorize my health care representative to make decisions in my best interest concerning withdrawal or withholding of health care. If at any time, based on my previously expressed preferences and the diagnosis and prognosis, my health care representative is satisfied that certain health care is not or would not be beneficial, or that such health care is or would be excessively burdensome, then my health care representative may express my will that such health care be withheld or withdrawn and may consent on my behalf that any or all health care be discontinued or not instituted, even if death may result.

My health care representative must try to discuss this decision with me. However, if I am unable to communicate, my health care representative may make such a decision for me, after consultation with my physician or physicians and other relevant health care givers. To the extent appropriate, my health care representative may also discuss this decision with my family and others, to the extent they are available.

Signature _____

Date _____

Witness name _____

Address _____

Telephone _____

Witness name _____

Address _____

Telephone _____

Subscribed, sworn to and acknowledged before me this _____ day of _____, 199___.

_____

Notary Public in and for the State of _____, _____ county. My commission expires _____.

Living Will Declaration

Declaration made this _____ day of _____ (month, year). I, _____, being at least eighteen (18) years old and of sound mind, willfully and voluntarily make known my desires that my dying shall not be artificially prolonged under the circumstances set forth below, and I declare:

If at any time I have an incurable injury, disease, or illness certified in writing to be a terminal condition by my attending physician, and my attending physician has determined that my death will occur within a short period of time, and the use of life-prolonging procedures would serve only to artificially prolong the dying process, I direct that such procedures be withheld or withdrawn, and that I be permitted to die naturally with only the provision of appropriate nutrition and hydration and the administration of medication and the performance of any medical procedure necessary to provide me with comfort care or to alleviate pain.

In the absence of my ability to give directions regarding the use of life-prolonging procedures, it is my intention that this declaration be honored by my family and physician as the final expression of my legal right to refuse medical or surgical treatment and accept the consequences of the refusal.

I understand the full import of this declaration.

Signed _____

_____
City, County, and State of Residence

The declarant has been personally known to me, and I believe (him/her) to be of sound mind. I did not sign the declarant's signature above for or at the direction of the declarant. I am not a parent, spouse, or child of the declarant. I am not entitled to any part of the declarant's estate or directly financially responsible for the declarant's medical care. I am competent and at least eighteen (18) years old.

Witness _____

Date _____

Address/telephone _____

Witness _____

Date _____

Address/telephone _____

IOWA

Declaration

If I should have an incurable or irreversible condition that will cause my death within a relatively short time, it is my desire that my life not be prolonged by administration of life-sustaining procedures. If my condition is terminal and I am unable to participate in decisions regarding my medical treatment, I direct my attending physician to withhold or withdraw procedures that merely prolong the dying process and are not necessary to my comfort or freedom from pain.

Signed this _____ day of _____, _____.
Signature:

_____

City, County and State of Residence:

_____

The declarant is known to me and voluntarily signed this document in my presence.

Witness _____

Address/Telephone _____

Witness _____

Address/Telephone _____

Durable Power of Attorney for Health Care Decisions General Statement of Authority Granted

I, _____, designate and appoint:

Name _____

Address: _____

Telephone Number: _____

to be my agent for health care decisions and pursuant to the language stated below, on my behalf to:

(1) Consent, refuse consent, or withdraw consent to any care, treatment, service or procedure to maintain, diagnose or treat a physical or mental condition, and to make decisions about organ donation, autopsy and disposition of the body;

(2) make all necessary arrangements at any hospital, psychiatric hospital or psychiatric treatment facility, hospice, nursing home or similar institution; to employ or discharge health care personnel to include physicians, psychiatrists, psychologists, dentists, nurses, therapists or any other person who is licensed, certified or otherwise authorized or permitted by the laws of this state to administer health care as the agent shall deem necessary for my physical, mental and emotional well being; and

(3) request, receive and review any information, verbal or written, regarding my personal affairs or physical or mental health including medical and hospital records and to execute any releases of other documents that may be required in order to obtain such information.

In exercising the grant of authority set forth above my agent for health care decisions shall:

_____

(Here may be inserted any special instructions or statement of the principal's desires to be followed by the agent in exercising the authority granted.)

LIMITATIONS OF AUTHORITY

(1) The powers of the agent herein shall be limited to the extent set out in writing in this durable power of attorney for health care decisions, and shall not include the power to revoke or invalidate any previously existing declaration made in accordance with the natural death act.

(2) The agent shall be prohibited from authorizing consent for the following items:

_____

_____

(3) This durable power of attorney for health care decisions shall be subject to the additional following limitations:

_____

_____

EFFECTIVE TIME

This power of attorney for health care decisions shall become effective if and when because of illness or injury, I become unable to make my own health care decisions, and shall remain in effect during such disability or incapacity.

REVOCATION

Any durable power of attorney for health care decisions I have previously made is hereby revoked.

(This durable power of attorney for health care decisions shall be revoked by an instrument in writing executed, witnessed or acknowledged in the same manner as required herein or set out another manner of revocation, if desired.

EXECUTION

Executed this _____, at _____, Kansas.

_____
Principal.

This document must be: (1) Witnessed by two individuals of lawful age who are not the agent, not related to the principal by blood, marriage or adoption, not entitled to any portion of principal's estate and not financially responsible for principal's health care; OR (2) acknowledged before a notary public.

Witness _____

Telephone _____

Address _____

Witness _____

Telephone _____

Address _____

(OR)

STATE OF _____)
) ss.
COUNTY OF _____)

This instrument was acknowledged before me on _____ by

_____

(Signature of notary public) _____

(Seal, if any)

My appointment expires: _____

Declaration

Declaration made this _____ day of _____ (month, year). I, _____, being of sound mind, willfully and voluntarily make known my desire that my dying shall not be artificially prolonged under the circumstances set forth below, do hereby declare:

If at any time I should have an incurable injury, disease, or illness certified to be a terminal condition by two physicians who have personally examined me, one of whom shall be my attending physician, and the physicians have determined that my death will occur whether or not life-sustaining procedures are utilized and where the application of life-sustaining procedures would serve only to artificially prolong the dying process, I direct that such procedures be withheld or withdrawn, and that I be permitted to die naturally with only the administration of medication or the performance of any medical procedure deemed necessary to provide me with comfort care.

In the absence of my ability to give directions regarding the use of such life-sustaining procedures, it is my intention that this declaration shall be honored by my family and physician(s) as the final expression of my legal right to refuse medical or surgical treatment and accept the consequences from such refusal.

I understand the full import of this declaration and I am emotionally and mentally competent to make this declaration.

Signed _____

City, County and State of Residence _____

_____

The declarant has been personally known to me and I believe him or her to be of sound mind. I did not sign the declarant's signature above for or at the direction of the declarant. I am not related to the declarant by blood or marriage, entitled to any portion of the estate of the declarant according to the laws of intestate succession or under any will of declarant or codicil thereto, or directly financially responsible for declarant's medical care.

Witness name _____

Address _____

Telephone _____

Witness name _____

Address _____

Telephone _____

Declaration

Declaration made this _____ day of _____, _____ (month, year). I, _____, willfully and voluntarily make known my desire that my dying shall not be artificially prolonged under the circumstances set forth below, and do hereby declare:

If at any time I should have a terminal condition and my attending and one (1) other physician in their discretion, have determined such condition is incurable and irreversible and will result in death within a relatively short time, and where the application of life-prolonging treatment would serve only to artificially prolong the dying process, I direct that such treatment be withheld or withdrawn, and that I be permitted to die naturally with only the administration of medication or the performance of any medical treatment deemed necessary to alleviate pain or for nutrition or hydration.

In the absence of my ability to give directions regarding the use of such life-prolonging treatment, it is my intention that this declaration shall be honored by my attending physician and my family as the final expression of my legal right to refuse medical or surgical treatment and I accept the consequences of such refusal.

If I have been diagnosed as pregnant and that diagnosis is known to my attending physician, this directive shall have no force or effect during the course of my pregnancy.

I understand the full import of this declaration and I am emotionally and mentally competent to make this declaration.

STATE OF KENTUCKY   )
) Sct.

COUNTY OF _____)

Before me, the undersigned authority, on this day personally appeared _____, Living Will Declarant, and _____ and _____, known to me to be witnesses whose names are each signed to the foregoing instrument, and all these persons being first duly sworn, _____, Living Will Declarant, declared to me and to the witnesses in my presence that the instrument is the Living Will Declaration of the declarant and that the declarant has willingly signed and that such declarant executed it as a free and voluntary act for the purposes therein expressed; and each of the witnesses stated to me, in the presence and hearing of the Living Will Declarant, that the declarant signed the declaration as witness and to the best of such witness's knowledge, the Living Will Declarant was eighteen (18) years of age or over, of sound mind and under no constraint or undue influence.

Living Will Declarant _____

Witness _____

Address/Telephone _____

Witness _____

Address/Telephone _____

Kentucky

Subscribed, sworn to and acknowledged before me by _____ and
_____, Living Will Declarant, and subscribed and sworn before me by
_____ and _____, witnesses, on this the
_____ day of _____ (year).

Notary Public State At Large _____

Date my commission expires _____

Declaration

Declaration made this _____ day of _____ (month, year).

I, _____, being of sound mind, willfully and voluntarily make known my desire that my dying shall not be artificially prolonged under the circumstances set forth below and do hereby declare:

If at any time I should have an incurable injury, disease or illness, or be in a continual profound comatose state with no reasonable chance of recovery, certified to be a terminal and irreversible condition by two physicians who have personally examined me, one of whom shall be my attending physician, and the physicians have determined that my death will occur whether or not life-sustaining procedures are utilized and where the application of life-sustaining procedure would serve only to prolong artificially the dying process, I direct that such procedures be withheld or written and that I be permitted to die naturally with only the administration of medication or the performance of any medical procedure deemed necessary to provide me with comfort care.

In the absence of my ability to give directions regarding the use of such life-sustaining procedures, it is my intention that this declaration shall be honored by my family and physician(s) as the final expression of my legal right to refuse medical or surgical treatment and accept the consequences from such refusal.

I understand the full import of this declaration and I am emotionally and mentally competent to make this declaration.

Signed _____

City, Parish and State of Residence _____

The declarant has been personally known to me and I believe him or her to be of sound mind.

Witness name _____

Address _____

Telephone _____

Witness name _____

Address _____

Telephone _____

MAINE

Declaration

If I am determined by my attending physician to be in a terminal condition or a persistent vegetative state, and I am no longer able to make or communicate decisions regarding my medical treatment, then I direct my attending physician to withhold or withdraw all life-sustaining treatment that is not necessary for my comfort or to alleviate pain.

Optional: If I am in a terminal condition or a persistent vegetative state, I want to receive nutrients and liquids provided through the use of tubes, intravenous procedures or similar medical interventions, even though other life-sustaining treatment is withheld or withdrawn.

Signature _____

NOTE: This optional provision must be signed to be effective. Otherwise, artificially administered nutrition and hydration may be withheld or withdrawn.

Signed this _____ day of _____, _____.

Signature _____

Address _____

Date of birth or social security number _____

The declarant voluntarily signed this writing in my presence.

Witness _____

Address/telephone _____

Witness _____

Address/telephone _____

NOTE: Maine law (18-A MRSA § 5-701) contains the following definitions of terms used in this declaration.

"Life-sustaining treatment" means any medical procedure or intervention that, when administered to a qualified patient, will serve only to prolong the process of dying. "Life-sustaining treatment" may include artificially administered nutrition and hydration, which is the provision of nutrients and liquids through the use of tubes, intravenous procedures or similar medical interventions.

"Terminal condition" means an incurable and irreversible condition that, without the administration of life-sustaining treatment, will, in the opinion of the attending physician, result in death within a relatively short time.

"Persistent vegetative state" means a state that occurs after coma in which the individual totally lacks higher cortical and cognitive function, but maintains vegetative brainstem processes, with no realistic possibility of recovery, as diagnosed in accordance with accepted medical standards. Vegetative brainstem processes may include one or more of the following: cycles of sleeping and waking, spontaneous eye opening and movements, some motor activity, vocalization, blood pressure, respiration and heart beat.

If you have questions about the meaning of this form, you are encouraged to seek the advice of a doctor or lawyer.

Declaration

On this _____ day of _____ (month, year), I _____, being of sound mind, willfully and voluntarily direct that my dying shall not be artificially prolonged under the circumstances set forth in this declaration:

If at any time I should have an incurable injury, disease, or illness certified to be a terminal condition by two (2) physicians who have personally examined me, one (1) of whom shall be my attending physician, and the physicians have determined that my death is imminent and will occur whether or not life-sustaining procedures are utilized and where the application of such procedures would serve only to artificially prolong the dying process, I direct that such procedures be withheld or withdrawn, and that I be permitted to die naturally with only the administration of medication, the administration of food and water, and the performance of any medical procedure that is necessary to provide comfort care or alleviate the pain. In the absence of my ability to give directions regarding the use of such life-sustaining procedures, it is my intention that this declaration shall be honored by my family and physician(s) as the final expression of my right to control my medical care and treatment.

I am legally competent to make this declaration, and I understand its full import.

Signed _____

Address _____

_____

Under penalty of perjury, we state that this declaration was signed by _____ in the presence of the undersigned who, at _____ request, in _____ presence, and in the presence of each other, have hereunto signed our names as witnesses this _____ day of _____ 19_____. Further, each of us, individually, states that: The declarant is known to me, and I believe the declarant to be of sound mind. I did not sign the declarant's signature to this decision. Based upon information and belief, I am not related to the declarant by blood or marriage, a creditor of the declarant, entitled to any portion of the estate of the declarant under any existing testamentary instrument of the declarant, entitled to any financial benefit by reason of the death of the declarant, financially or otherwise responsible for the declarant's medical care, nor an employee of any such person or institution.

Witness Name _____

Address/Telephone _____

Witness Name _____

Address/Telephone _____

MICHIGAN —————————————————————

Agent's Acceptance

I agree to act as the health care agent for (name) _____. I understand that:

(a) This designation shall not become effective unless the patient is unable to participate in medical treatment decisions.

(b) A patient advocate shall not exercise powers concerning the patient's care, custody, and medical treatment that the patient, if the patient were able to participate in the decision, could not have exercised on his or her own behalf.

(c) This designation cannot be used to make a medical treatment decision to withhold or withdraw treatment from a patient who is pregnant that would result in the pregnant patient's death.

(d) A patient advocate may make a decision to withhold or withdraw treatment which would allow a patient to die only if the patient has expressed in a clear and convincing manner that the patient advocate is authorized to make such a decision, and that the patient acknowledges that such a decision could or would allow the patient's death.

(e) A patient advocate shall not receive compensation for the performance of his or her authority, rights, and responsibilities, but a patient advocate may be reimbursed for actual and necessary expenses incurred in the performance of his or her authority, rights, and responsibilities.

(f) A patient advocate shall act in accordance with the standards of care applicable to fiduciaries when acting for the patient and shall act consistent with the patient's best interests. The known desires of the patient expressed or evidenced while the patient is able to participate in medical treatment decisions are presumed to be in the patient's best interests.

(g) A patient may revoke his or her designation at any time and in any manner sufficient to communicate an intent to revoke.

(h) A patient advocate may revoke his or her acceptance to the designation at any time and in any manner sufficient to communicate an intent to revoke.

(i) A patient admitted to a health facility or agency has the rights enumerated in section 20201 of the public health code, Act No. 368 of the Public Acts of 1978, being section 333.20201 of the Michigan Compiled Laws.

Name _____

Date _____

Health Care Declaration

Notice:

This is an important legal document. Before signing this document, you should know these important facts:

(a) This document gives your health care providers or your designated proxy the power and guidance to make health care decisions according to your wishes when you are in a terminal condition and cannot do so. This document may include what kind of treatment you want or do not want and under what circumstances you want these decisions to be made. You may state where you want or do not want to receive any treatment.

(b) If you name a proxy in this document and that person agrees to serve as your proxy, that person has a duty to act consistently with your wishes. If the proxy does not know your wishes, the proxy has the duty to act in your best interests. If you do not name a proxy, your health care providers have a duty to act consistently with your instructions or tell you that they are unwilling to do so.

(c) This document will remain valid and in effect until and unless you amend or revoke it. Review this document periodically to make sure it continues to reflect your preferences. You may amend or revoke the declaration at any time by notifying your health care providers.

(d) Your named proxy has the same right as you have to examine your medical records and to consent to their disclosure for purposes related to your health care or insurance unless you limit this right in this document.

(e) If there is anything in this document that you do not understand, you should ask for professional help to have it explained to you.

TO MY FAMILY, DOCTORS, AND ALL THOSE CONCERNED WITH MY CARE:

I, _____, born on (birthdate) _____ being an adult of sound mind, willfully and voluntarily make this statement as a directive to be followed if I am in a terminal condition and become unable to participate in decisions regarding my health care. I understand that my health care providers are legally bound to act consistently with my wishes, within the limits of reasonable medical practice and other applicable law. I also understand that I have the right to make medical and health care decisions for myself as long as I am able to do so and to revoke this declaration at any time.

(1) The following are my feelings and wishes regarding my health care (you may state the circumstances under which this declaration applies):

_____

_____

_____

_____

(2) I particularly want to have all appropriate health care that will help in the following ways (you may give instructions for care you do want):

_____

_____

_____

_____

(3) I particularly do not want the following (you may list specific treatment you do not want in certain circumstances):

_____

_____

_____

_____

(4) I particularly want to have the following kinds of life-sustaining treatment if I am diagnosed to have a terminal condition (you may list the specific types of life-sustaining treatment that you do want if you have a terminal condition):

_____

_____

_____

_____

(5) I particularly do not want the following kinds of life-sustaining treatment if I am diagnosed to have a terminal condition (you may list the specific types of life-sustaining treatment that you do not want if you have a terminal condition):

_____

_____

_____

_____

(6) I recognize that if I reject artificially administered sustenance, then I may die of dehydration or malnutrition rather than from my illness or injury. The following are my feelings and wishes regarding artificially administered sustenance should I have a terminal condition (you may indicate whether you wish to receive food and fluids given to you in some other way than by mouth if you have a terminal condition):

_____

_____

_____

_____

(7) Thoughts I feel are relevant to my instructions. (You may, but need not, give your religious beliefs, philosophy, or other personal values that you feel are important. You may also state preferences concerning the location of your care.)

_____

_____

_____

_____

(8) Proxy Designation. (If you wish, you may name someone to see that your wishes are carried out, but you do not have to do this. You may also name a proxy without including specific instructions regarding your care. If you name a proxy, you should discuss your wishes with that person.)

If I become unable to communicate my instructions, I designate the following person(s) to act on my behalf consistently with my instructions, if any, as stated in this document. Unless I write instructions that limit my proxy's authority, my proxy has full power and authority to make health care decisions for me. If a guardian or conservator of the person is to be appointed for me, I nominate my proxy named in this document to act as guardian or conservator of my person.

Name: _____

Address: _____

Phone Number: _____

Relationship: (If any) _____

If the person I have named above refuses or is unable or unavailable to act on my behalf, or if I revoke that person's authority to act as my proxy, I authorize the following person to do so:

Name: _____

Address: _____

Phone Number: _____

Relationship: (If any) _____

I understand that I have the right to revoke the appointment of the persons named above to act on my behalf at any time by communicating that decision to the proxy or my health care provider.

I (have) (have not) agreed in another document or on another form to donate some or all of my organs when I die.

DATE: _____

SIGNED: _____

STATE OF _____

COUNTY OF _____

Subscribed, sworn to, and acknowledged before me by _____
on this _____ day of _____, 19___.

NOTARY PUBLIC

Minnesota

OR

(Sign and date here in the presence of two adult witnesses, neither of whom is entitled to any part of your estate under a will or by operation of law, and neither of whom is your proxy.)

I certify that the declarant voluntarily signed this declaration in my presence and that the declarant is personally known to me. I am not named as a proxy by the declaration, and to the best of my knowledge, I am not entitled to any part of the estate of the declarant under a will or by operation of law.

Witness _____

Address/telephone _____

Witness _____

Address/telephone _____

Reminder: Keep the signed original with your personal papers.
Give signed copies to your doctors, family, and proxy.

Notice to Person Executing This Document—Health Care Power of Attorney

This is an important legal document. Before executing this document, you should know these important facts:

This document gives the person you designate as the attorney in fact (your agent) the power to make health care decisions for you. This power exists only as to those health care decisions to which you are unable to give informed consent. The attorney in fact must act consistently with your desires as stated in this document or otherwise made known.

Except as you otherwise specify in this document, this document gives your agent the power to consent to your doctor not giving treatment or stopping treatment necessary to keep you alive.

Notwithstanding this document, you have the right to make medical and other health care decisions for yourself so long as you can give informed consent with respect to the particular decision. In addition, no treatment may be given to you over your objection, and health care necessary to keep you alive may not be stopped or withheld if you object at the time.

The document gives your agent authority to consent, to refuse to consent or to withdraw consent to any care, treatment, service or procedure to maintain, diagnose or treat a physical or mental condition. This power is subject to any statement of your desires and any limitations that you include in this document. You may state in this document any types of treatment that you do not desire. In addition, a court can take away the power of your agent to make health care decisions for you if your agent (a) authorizes anything that is illegal, (b) acts contrary to your known desires, or (c) where your desires are not known, does anything that is clearly contrary to your best interests.

You have the right to revoke the authority of your agent by notifying your agent or your treating doctor, hospital or other health care provider in writing of the revocation.

Your agent has the right to examine your medical records and to consent to this disclosure unless you limit this right in this document.

Unless you otherwise specify in this document, this document gives your agent the power after you die to (a) authorize an autopsy, (b) donate your body or parts thereof for transplant or for educational, therapeutic or scientific purposes, and (c) direct the disposition of your remains.

If there is anything in this document that you do not understand you should ask your lawyer to explain it to you.

This power of attorney will not be valid for making health care decisions unless it is either (a) signed by two (2) qualified adult witnesses who are personally known to you and who are present when you sign or acknowledge your signature or (b) acknowledged before a notary public in the state.

I have read this notice and I understand it.

Signature _____

Date _____

MISSISSIPPI _____

Declaration

Declaration made on _____ (date) by _____ (person's name) of
_____ (address), _____ (Social Security Number).
    I, _____, being of sound mind, declare that if at any time I should suffer a terminal physical condition which causes me severe distress or unconsciousness, and my physician, with the concurrence of two (2) other physicians, believes that there is no expectation of my regaining consciousness or a state of health that is meaningful to me and but for the use of life-sustaining mechanisms my death would be imminent, I desire that the mechanisms be withdrawn so that I may die naturally. However, if I have been diagnosed as pregnant and that diagnosis is known to my physician, this declaration shall have no force or effect during the course of my pregnancy. I further declare that this declaration shall be honored by my family and my physician as the final expression of my desires concerning the manner in which I die.

SIGNED _____

I hereby witness this declaration and attest that:
(1) I personally know the Declarant and believe the Declarant to be of sound mind.
(2) To the best of my knowledge, at the time of the execution of this declaration, I:
(a) Am not related to the Declarant by blood or marriage,
(b) Do not have any claim on the estate of the Declarant,
(c) Am not entitled to any portion of the Declarant's estate by any will or by operation of law, and
(d) Am not a physician attending the Declarant or a person employed by a physician attending the Declarant.

WITNESS _____
ADDRESS/TELEPHONE _____
SOCIAL SECURITY NUMBER _____

WITNESS _____
ADDRESS/TELEPHONE _____
SOCIAL SECURITY NUMBER _____

This document must be filed with the bureau of vital statistics of the state board of health.

Revocation of Declaration

(1) A declaration executed as provided in section 41-41-107 may be revoked by a revocation signed by the declarant and at least two (2) persons who witnessed the declarant's execution of the revocation which shall be in substantially the following form:

On _____ (date), I, _____, (person's name), of _____ (address), _____ (Social Security Number), being of sound mind, revoke the declaration made on _____ (date declaration made) regarding the manner in which I die.

SIGNED _____

I hereby witness this revocation and attest that:

(1) I personally know the maker of this revocation and believe the maker of this revocation to be of sound mind.

(2) To the best of my knowledge, at the time of the execution of this revocation, I:

(a) Am not related to the maker of this revocation by blood or marriage,

(b) Do not have any claim on the estate of the maker of this revocation,

(c) Am not entitled to any portion of the estate of the maker of this revocation by any will or by operation of law, and

(d) Am not a physician attending the maker of the revocation or a person employed by a physician attending the maker of this revocation.

WITNESS _____

ADDRESS/TELEPHONE _____

SOCIAL SECURITY NUMBER _____

WITNESS _____

ADDRESS/TELEPHONE _____

SOCIAL SECURITY NUMBER _____

This document must be filed with the bureau of vital statistics of the state board of health.

Declaration

I have the primary right to make my own decisions concerning treatment that might unduly prolong the dying process. By this declaration I express to my physician, family and friends my intent. If I should have a terminal condition it is my desire that my dying not be prolonged by administration of death-prolonging procedures. If my condition is terminal and I am unable to participate in decisions regarding my medical treatment, I direct my attending physician to withhold or withdraw medical procedures that merely prolong the dying process and are not necessary to my comfort or to alleviate pain. It is not my intent to authorize affirmative or deliberate acts or omissions to shorten my life rather only to permit the natural process of dying.

Signed this _____ day of _____, 199___.

Signature _____

City, County and State of residence _____

The declarant is known to me, is eighteen years of age or older, of sound mind and voluntarily signed this document in my presence.

Witness _____

Address _____

Telephone _____

Witness _____

Address _____

Telephone _____

MONTANA ‎——————————————————

Declaration

If I should have an incurable or irreversible condition that, without the administration of life-sustaining treatment, will, in the opinion of my attending physician, cause my death within a relatively short time and I am no longer able to make decisions regarding my medical treatment, I direct my attending physician, pursuant to the Montana Rights of the Terminally Ill Act, to withhold or withdraw treatment that only prolongs the process of dying and is not necessary to my comfort or to alleviate pain.

    Signed this _____ day of _____, 199___.

Signature _____

City, County, and State of Residence _____

The declarant voluntarily signed this document in my presence.

Witness _____

Address/telephone _____

Witness _____

Address/telephone _____

Power of Attorney for Health Care

I appoint _____, whose address is _____, and whose telephone number is _____, as my attorney in fact for health care. I appoint _____, whose address is _____, and whose telephone number is _____, as my successor attorney in fact for health care. I authorize my attorney in fact appointed by this document to make health care decisions for me when I am determined to be incapable of making my own health care decisions. I have read the warning which accompanies this document and understand the consequences of executing a power of attorney for health care.

I direct that my attorney in fact comply with the following instructions or limitations:

_____

_____

I direct that my attorney in fact comply with the following instructions on life-sustaining treatment: (optional)

_____

_____

I direct that my attorney in fact comply with the following instructions on artificially administered nutrition and hydration: (optional)

_____

_____

(Signature of person making designation/date) _____

DECLARATION OF WITNESSES

We declare that the principal is personally known to us, that the principal signed or acknowledged his or her signature on this power of attorney for health care in our presence, that the principal appears to be of sound mind and not under duress or undue influence, and that neither of us nor the principal's attending physician is the person appointed as attorney in fact by this document.

Witnessed By:

(Signature of Witness/Date) _____

(Printed Name of Witness) _____

(Address) _____

(Telephone) _____

Nebraska

(Signature of Witness/Date) _____

(Printed Name of Witness) _____

(Address) _____

(Telephone) _____

WARNING TO PERSON EXECUTING A POWER OF ATTORNEY
FOR HEALTH CARE

This is an important legal document. It creates a power of attorney for health care. Before signing this document you should know these important facts:

(a) This document gives the person you designate as your attorney in fact the power to make health care decisions for you when you are determined to be incapable. Although not necessary and neither encouraged nor discouraged, you may wish to state instructions or wishes and limit the authority of your attorney in fact;

(b) Subject to the limitation stated in subdivision (d) of this document, the person you designate as your attorney in fact has a duty to act consistently with your desires as stated in this document or otherwise made known by you or, if your desires are unknown, to act in a manner consistent with your best interests. The person you designate in this document does, however, have the right to withdraw from this duty at any time;

(c) You may specify that any determination that you are incapable of making health care decisions must be confirmed by a second physician;

(d) The person you designate as your attorney in fact will not have the authority to consent to the withholding or withdrawal of life-sustaining procedures or of artificially administered nutrition or hydration unless you give him or her that authority in this power of attorney for health care or in some other clear and convincing manner;

(e) This power of attorney for health care should be reviewed periodically. It will continue in effect indefinitely unless you exercise your right to revoke it. You have the right to revoke this power of attorney at any time while you are competent by notifying the attorney in fact or your health care provider of the revocation orally or in writing;

(f) Despite any provisions in this power of attorney for health care, you have the right to make health care decisions for yourself as long as you are not incapable of making those decisions; and

(g) If there is anything in this power of attorney for health care you do not understand, you should seek legal advice. This power of attorney for health care will not be valid for making health care decisions unless it is signed by two qualified witnesses who are personally known to you and who are present when you sign or acknowledge your signature.

Declaration

If I should lapse into a persistent vegetative state or have an incurable and irreversible condition that, without the administration of life-sustaining treatment, will, in the opinion of my attending physician, cause my death within a relatively short time and I am no longer able to make decisions regarding my medical treatment, I direct my attending physician, pursuant to the Rights of the Terminally Ill Act, to withhold or withdraw life sustaining treatment that is not necessary for my comfort or to alleviate pain.

Signed this _____ day of _____, 199___.

Signature _____

Address _____

The declarant voluntarily signed this writing in my presence.

Witness _____

Address _____

Telephone _____

Witness _____

Address _____

Telephone _____

Or

The declarant voluntarily signed this writing in my presence.

Notary Public _____

Durable Power of Attorney for Health Care Decisions

WARNING TO PERSON EXECUTING THIS DOCUMENT

THIS IS AN IMPORTANT LEGAL DOCUMENT. IT CREATES A DURABLE POWER OF ATTORNEY FOR HEALTH CARE. BEFORE EXECUTING THIS DOCUMENT, YOU SHOULD KNOW THESE IMPORTANT FACTS:

1. THIS DOCUMENT GIVES THE PERSON YOU DESIGNATE AS YOUR ATTORNEY-IN-FACT THE POWER TO MAKE HEALTH CARE DECISIONS FOR YOU. THIS POWER IS SUBJECT TO ANY LIMITATIONS OR STATEMENT OF YOUR DESIRES THAT YOU INCLUDE IN THIS DOCUMENT. THE POWER TO MAKE HEALTH CARE DECISIONS FOR YOU MAY INCLUDE CONSENT, REFUSAL OF CONSENT, OR WITHDRAWAL OF CONSENT TO ANY CARE, TREATMENT, SERVICE, OR PROCEDURE TO MAINTAIN, DIAGNOSE, OR TREAT A PHYSICAL OR MENTAL CONDITION. YOU MAY STATE IN THIS DOCUMENT ANY TYPES OF TREATMENT OR PLACEMENTS THAT YOU DO NOT DESIRE.

2. THE PERSON YOU DESIGNATE IN THIS DOCUMENT HAS A DUTY TO ACT CONSISTENT WITH YOUR DESIRES AS STATED IN THIS DOCUMENT OR OTHERWISE MADE KNOWN OR, IF YOUR DESIRES ARE UNKNOWN, TO ACT IN YOUR BEST INTERESTS.

3. EXCEPT AS YOU OTHERWISE SPECIFY IN THIS DOCUMENT, THE POWER OF THE PERSON YOU DESIGNATE TO MAKE HEALTH CARE DECISIONS FOR YOU MAY INCLUDE THE POWER TO CONSENT TO YOUR DOCTOR NOT GIVING TREATMENT OR STOPPING TREATMENT WHICH WOULD KEEP YOU ALIVE.

4. UNLESS YOU SPECIFY A SHORTER PERIOD IN THIS DOCUMENT, THIS POWER WILL EXIST INDEFINITELY FROM THE DATE YOU EXECUTE THIS DOCUMENT AND, IF YOU ARE UNABLE TO MAKE HEALTH CARE DECISIONS FOR YOURSELF, THIS POWER WILL CONTINUE TO EXIST UNTIL THE TIME WHEN YOU BECOME ABLE TO MAKE HEALTH CARE DECISIONS FOR YOURSELF.

5. NOTWITHSTANDING THIS DOCUMENT, YOU HAVE THE RIGHT TO MAKE MEDICAL AND OTHER HEALTH CARE DECISIONS FOR YOURSELF SO LONG AS YOU CAN GIVE INFORMED CONSENT WITH RESPECT TO THE PARTICULAR DECISION. IN ADDITION, NO TREATMENT MAY BE GIVEN TO YOU OVER YOUR OBJECTION, AND HEALTH CARE NECESSARY TO KEEP YOU ALIVE MAY NOT BE STOPPED IF YOU OBJECT.

6. YOU HAVE THE RIGHT TO REVOKE THE APPOINTMENT OF THE PERSON DESIGNATED IN THIS DOCUMENT TO MAKE HEALTH CARE DECISIONS FOR YOU BY NOTIFYING THAT PERSON OF THE REVOCATION ORALLY OR IN WRITING.

7. YOU HAVE THE RIGHT TO REVOKE THE AUTHORITY GRANTED TO THE PERSON DESIGNATED IN THIS DOCUMENT TO MAKE HEALTH CARE DECISIONS FOR YOU BY NOTIFYING THE TREATING PHYSICIAN, HOSPITAL, OR OTHER PROVIDER OF HEALTH CARE ORALLY OR IN WRITING.

8. THE PERSON DESIGNATED IN THIS DOCUMENT TO MAKE HEALTH CARE DECISIONS FOR YOU HAS THE RIGHT TO EXAMINE YOUR MEDICAL RECORDS AND TO CONSENT TO THEIR DISCLOSURE UNLESS YOU LIMIT THIS RIGHT IN THIS DOCUMENT.

Nevada

9. THIS DOCUMENT REVOKES ANY PRIOR DURABLE POWER OF ATTORNEY FOR HEALTH CARE.

10. IF THERE IS ANYTHING IN THIS DOCUMENT THAT YOU DO NOT UNDERSTAND, YOU SHOULD ASK A LAWYER TO EXPLAIN IT TO YOU.

1. DESIGNATION OF HEALTH CARE AGENT.

I, _____ (insert your name) do hereby designate and appoint:

Name: _____

Address: _____

Telephone Number: _____

as my attorney-in-fact to make health care decisions for me as authorized in this document.

(Insert the name and address of the person you wish to designate as your attorney-in-fact to make health care decisions for you. None of the following may be designated as your attorney-in-fact: (1) your treating provider of health care, (2) an employee of your treating provider of health care, (3) an operator of a health care facility, or (4) an employee of an operator of a health care facility.)

2. CREATION OF DURABLE POWER OF ATTORNEY FOR HEALTH CARE.

By this document I intend to create a durable power of attorney by appointing the person designated above to make health care decisions for me. This power of attorney shall not be affected by my subsequent incapacity.

3. GENERAL STATEMENT OF AUTHORITY GRANTED.

In the event that I am incapable of giving informed consent with respect to health care decisions, I hereby grant to the attorney-in-fact named above full power and authority to make health care decisions for me before, or after my death, including: consent, refusal of consent, or withdrawal of consent to any care, treatment, service, or procedure to maintain, diagnose, or treat a physical or mental condition, subject only to the limitations and special provisions, if any, set forth in paragraph 4 or 6.

4. SPECIAL PROVISIONS AND LIMITATIONS.

(Your attorney-in-fact is not permitted to consent to any of the following: commitment to or placement in a mental health treatment facility, convulsive treatment, psychosurgery, sterilization, or abortion. If there are any other types of treatment or placement that you do not want your attorney-in-fact's authority to give consent for or other restrictions you wish to place on his or her attorney-in-fact's authority, you should list them in the space below. If you do not write any limitations, your attorney-in-fact will have the broad powers to make health care decisions on your behalf which are set forth in paragraph 3, except to the extent that there are limits provided by law.)

In exercising the authority under this durable power of attorney for health care, the authority of my attorney-in-fact is subject to the following special provisions and limitations:

_____

_____

_____

_____

5. DURATION.

I understand that this power of attorney will exist indefinitely from the date I execute this document unless I establish a shorter time. If I am unable to make health care decisions for myself when this power of attorney expires, the authority I have granted my attorney-in-fact will continue to exist until the time when I become able to make health care decisions for myself.

(IF APPLICABLE)
I wish to have this power of attorney end on the following
date: _____

6. STATEMENT OF DESIRES.

(With respect to decisions to withhold or withdraw life-sustaining treatment, your attorney-in-fact must make health care decisions that are consistent with your known desires. You can, but are not required to, indicate your desires below. If your desires are unknown, your attorney-in-fact has the duty to act in your best interests; and, under some circumstances, a judicial proceeding may be necessary so that a court can determine the health care decision that is in your best interests. If you wish to indicate your desires, you may INITIAL the statement or statements that reflect your desires and/or write your own statements in the space below.)

(If the statement reflects your desires, initial the box next to the statement.)

1. I desire that my life be prolonged to the greatest extent possible, without regard to my condition, the chances I have for recovery or long-term survival, or the cost of the procedures.

2. If I am in a coma which my doctors have reasonably concluded is irreversible, I desire that life-sustaining or prolonging treatments not be used. (Also should utilize provisions of NRS 449.540 to 449.690, inclusive, and sections 2 to 12, inclusive, of this act if this subparagraph is initialed.)

3. If I have an incurable or terminal condition or illness and no reasonable hope of long-term recovery or survival, I desire that life sustaining or prolonging treatments not be used. (Also should utilize provisions of NRS 449.540 to 449.690, inclusive, and sections 2 to 12, inclusive, of this act if this subparagraph is initialed.)

4. I direct my attending physician not to withhold or withdraw artificial nutrition and hydration by way of the gastro-intestinal tract if such a withholding or withdrawal would result in my death by starvation or dehydration.

5. I do not desire treatment to be provided and/or continued if the burdens of the treatment outweigh the expected benefits. My attorney-in-fact is to consider the relief of suffering, the preservation or restoration of functioning, and the quality as well as the extent of the possible extension of my life.

(If you wish to change your answer, you may do so by drawing an "X" through the answer you do not want, and circling the answer you prefer.)

Other or Additional Statements of Desires: _____

_____

_____

_____

_____

7. DESIGNATION OF ALTERNATE ATTORNEY-IN-FACT.

(Your are not required to designate any alternative attorney-in-fact but you may do so. Any alternative attorney-in-fact you designate will be able to make the same health care decisions as the attorney-in-fact designated in paragraph 1, page 2, in the event that he or she is unable or unwilling to act as your attorney-in-fact. Also, if the attorney-in-fact designated in paragraph 1 is your spouse, his or her designation as your attorney-in-fact is automatically revoked by law if your marriage is dissolved.)

If the person designated in paragraph 1 as my attorney-in-fact is unable to make health care decisions for me, then I designate the following persons to serve as my attorney-in-fact to make health care decisions for me as authorized in this document, such persons to serve in the order listed below:

A. First Alternative Attorney-in-fact

Name: _____

Address: _____

_____

Telephone Number: _____

B. Second Alternative Attorney-in-fact

Name: _____

Address: _____

_____

Telephone Number: _____

8. PRIOR DESIGNATIONS REVOKED. I revoke any prior durable power of attorney for health care.

(YOU MUST DATE AND SIGN THIS POWER OF ATTORNEY)

I sign my name to this Durable Power of Attorney for Health care on _____ (date) at _____ (city), _____ (state)

(Signature) _____

(THIS POWER OF ATTORNEY WILL NOT BE VALID FOR MAKING HEALTH CARE DECISIONS UNLESS IT IS EITHER (1) SIGNED BY AT LEAST TWO QUALIFIED WITNESSES WHO ARE PERSONALLY KNOWN TO YOU AND WHO ARE PRESENT WHEN YOU SIGN OR ACKNOWLEDGE YOUR SIGNATURE OR (2) ACKNOWLEDGED BEFORE A NOTARY PUBLIC.)

CERTIFICATE OF ACKNOWLEDGMENT OF NOTARY PUBLIC

(You may use acknowledgment before a notary public instead of the statement of witnesses.)

State of Nevada   }

} ss.

County of _____ }

On this _____ day of _____, in the year _____, before me, _____ (here insert name of notary public) personally appeared _____ (here insert name of principal) personally known to me (or proved to me on the basis of satisfactory evidence) to be the person whose name is subscribed to this instrument, and acknowledged that he or she executed it. I declare under penalty of perjury that the person whose name is ascribed to this instrument appears to be of sound mind and under no duress, fraud, or undue influence.

NOTARY SEAL   (Signature of Notary Public) _____

STATEMENT OF WITNESSES

(You should carefully read and follow this witnessing procedure. This document will not be valid unless you comply with the witnessing procedure. If you elect to use witnesses instead of having this document notarized you must use two qualified adult witnesses. None of the following may be used as a witness: (1) a person you designate as the attorney-in-fact, (2) a provider of health care, (3) an employee of a provider of health care, (4) the operator of a health care facility, (5) an employee of an operator of a health care facility. At least one of the witnesses must make the additional declaration set out following the place where the witnesses sign.)

I declare under penalty of perjury that the principal is personally known to me, that the principal signed or acknowledged this durable power of attorney in my presence, that the principal appears to be of sound mind and under no duress, fraud, or undue influence, that I am not the person appointed as attorney-in-fact by this document, and that I am not a provider of health care, an employee of a provider of health care, the operator of a community care facility, nor an employee of an operator of a health care facility.

Signature: _____

Print Name: _____

Date: _____

Residence Address: _____

_____

_____

Signature: _____

Print Name: _____

Date: _____

Residence Address: _____

_____

_____

(AT LEAST ONE OF THE ABOVE WITNESSES MUST ALSO
SIGN THE FOLLOWING DECLARATION.)

I declare under penalty of perjury that I am not related to the principal by blood, marriage, or adoption, and to the best of my knowledge I am not entitled to any part of the estate of the principal upon the death of the principal under a will now existing or by operation of law.

Signature: _____

Signature: _____

Names: _____

Print Name: _____

Date: _____

Address: _____

_____

_____

COPIES: You should retain an executed copy of this document and give one to your attorney-in-fact. The power of attorney should be available so a copy may be given to your providers of health care.

Declaration

If I should have an incurable and irreversible condition that, without the administration of life-sustaining treatment, will, in the opinion of my attending physician, cause my death within a relatively short time, and I am no longer able to make decisions regarding my medical treatment, I direct my attending physician, pursuant to NRS 449.540 to 449.690, inclusive, and sections 2 to 12, inclusive, of this act, to withhold or withdraw treatment that only prolongs the process of dying and is not necessary for my comfort or to alleviate pain.

    If you wish to include this statement, you must INITIAL the statement in the box provided.

    (If the statement reflects your desires, initial the box next to the statement.)

    I direct my attending physician not to withhold or withdraw artificial nutrition and hydration by way of the gastro-intestinal tract if such a withholding or withdrawal would result in my death by starvation or dehydration.

    Signed this _____ day of _____, _____.

Signature _____

Address _____

The declarant voluntarily signed this writing in my presence.

Witness _____

Address/telephone _____

Witness _____

Address/telephone _____

Information Concerning the Durable Power of Attorney for Health Care

THIS IS AN IMPORTANT LEGAL DOCUMENT. BEFORE SIGNING THIS DOCUMENT YOU SHOULD KNOW THESE IMPORTANT FACTS:

Except to the extent you state otherwise, this document gives the person you name as your agent the authority to make any and all health care decisions for you when you are no longer capable of making them yourself. "Health care" means any treatment, service or procedure to maintain, diagnose or treat your physical or mental condition. Your agent, therefore, can have the power to make a broad range of health care decisions for you. Your agent may consent, refuse to consent, or withdraw consent to medical treatment and may make decisions about withdrawing or withholding life-sustaining treatment. Your agent cannot consent or direct any of the following: commitment to a state institution, sterilization, or termination of treatment if you are pregnant and if the withdrawal of that treatment is deemed likely to terminate the pregnancy unless the failure to withhold the treatment will be physically harmful to you or prolong severe pain which cannot be alleviated by medication.

You may state in this document any treatment you do not desire, except as stated above, or treatment you want to be sure you receive. Your agent's authority will begin when your doctor certifies that you lack the capacity to make health care decisions. If for moral or religious reasons you do not wish to be treated by a doctor or examined by a doctor for the certification that you lack capacity, you must say so in the document and name a person to be able to certify your lack of capacity. That person may not be your agent or alternate agent or any person ineligible to be your agent. You may attach additional pages if you need more space to complete your statement.

If you want to give your agent authority to withhold or withdraw the artificial providing of nutrition and fluids, your document must say so. Otherwise, your agent will not be able to direct that. Under no conditions will your agent be able to direct the withholding of food and drink for you to eat and drink normally.

Your agent will be obligated to follow your instructions when making decisions on your behalf. Unless you state otherwise, your agent will have the same authority to make decisions about your health care as you would have had if made consistent with state law.

It is important that you discuss this document with your physician or other health care providers before you sign it to make sure that you understand the nature and range of decisions which may be made on your behalf. If you do not have a physician, you should talk with someone else who is knowledgeable about these issues and can answer your questions. You do not need a lawyer's assistance to complete this document, but if there is anything in this document that you do not understand, you should ask a lawyer to explain it to you.

The person you appoint as agent should be someone you know and trust and must be at least 18 years old. If you appoint your health or residential care provider (e.g. your physician, or an employee of a home health agency, hospital, nursing home, or residential care home, other than a relative), that person will have to choose between acting as your agent or as your health or residential care provider; the law does not permit a person to do both at the same time.

You should inform the person you appoint that you want him or her to be your health care agent. You should discuss this document with your agent and your physician and give each a signed copy. You should indicate on the document itself the people and institutions who will have signed copies. Your agent will not be liable for health care decisions made in good faith on your behalf.

Even after you have signed this document, you have the right to make health care decisions for yourself as long as you are able to do so, and treatment cannot be given to you or stopped over your objection. You have the right to revoke the authority granted to your agent by informing him or her or your health care provider orally or in writing.

This document may not be changed or modified. If you want to make changes in the document you must make an entirely new one.

You should consider designating an alternate agent in the event that your agent is unwilling, unable, unavailable, or ineligible to act as your agent. Any alternate agent you designate will have the same authority to make health care decisions for you.

THIS POWER OF ATTORNEY WILL NOT BE VALID UNLESS IT IS SIGNED IN THE PRESENCE OF TWO (2) OR MORE QUALIFIED WITNESSES WHO MUST BOTH BE PRESENT WHEN YOU SIGN AND AC-KNOWLEDGE YOUR SIGNATURE. THE FOLLOWING PERSONS MAY NOT ACT AS WITNESSES:

—the person you have designated as your agent;

—your spouse;

—your lawful heirs or beneficiaries named in your will or a deed;

ONLY ONE OF THE TWO WITNESSES MAY BE YOUR HEALTH OR RESIDENTIAL CARE PROVIDER OR ONE OF THEIR EMPLOYEES.

DURABLE POWER OF ATTORNEY FOR HEALTH CARE

I, _____, hereby appoint _____ of _____ as my agent to make any and all health care decisions for me, except to the extent I state otherwise in this document or as prohibited by law. This durable power of attorney for health care shall take effect in the event I become unable to make my own health care decisions.

STATEMENT OF DESIRES, SPECIAL PROVISIONS, AND LIMITATIONS REGARDING HEALTH CARE DECISIONS.

For your convenience in expressing your wishes, some general statements concerning the withholding or removal of life-sustaining treatment are set forth below. (Life-sustaining treatment is defined as proce-dures without which a person would die, such as but not limited to the following: cardiopulmonary resuscitation, mechanical respiration, kidney dialysis or the use of other external mechanical and tech-nological devices, drugs to maintain blood pressure, blood transfusions, and antibiotics.) There is also a section which allows you to set forth specific directions for these or other matters. If you wish you may indicate your agreement or disagreement with any of the following statements and give your agent power to act in those specific circumstances.

1. If I become permanently incompetent to make health care decisions, and if I am also suffering from a terminal illness, I authorize my agent to direct that life-sustaining treatment be discontinued. (YES) (NO) (Circle your choice and initial beneath it.)

2. Whether terminally ill or not, if I become permanently unconscious I authorize my agent to direct that life-sustaining treatment be discontinued. (YES) (NO) (Circle your choice and initial beneath it.)

3. I realize that situations could arise in which the only way to allow me to die would be to discontinue artificial feeding (artificial nutrition and hydration). In carrying out any instructions I have given above in #1 or #2 or any instructions I may write in #4 below, I authorize my agent to direct that (circle your choice of (a) or (b) and initial beside it):

(a) artificial nutrition and hydration not to be started or, if started, be discontinued,

-or-

(b) although all other forms of life-sustaining treatment be withdrawn, artificial nutrition and hydra-tion continue to be given to me. (If you fail to complete item 3, your agent will not have the power to direct the withdrawal of artificial nutrition and hydration.)

4. Here you may include any specific desires or limitations you deem appropriate, such as when or what life-sustaining treatment you would want used or withheld, or instructions about refusing any specific types of treatment that are inconsistent with your religious beliefs or unacceptable to you for any other reason. You may leave this question blank if you desire.

_____

_____

_____

_____

_____

(attach additional pages as necessary)

In the event the person I appoint above is unable, unwilling or unavailable, or ineligible to act as my health care agent, I hereby appoint _____ of _____ as alternate agent.

I hereby acknowledge that I have been provided with a disclosure statement explaining the effect of this document. I have read and understand the information contained in the disclosure statement.

The original of this document will be kept at _____ and the following persons and institutions will have signed copies:

_____

_____

_____

In witness whereof, I have hereunto signed my name this _____ day of _____, 19_____

Signature _____

I declare that the principal appears to be of sound mind and free from duress at the time the durable power of attorney for health care is signed and that the principal has affirmed that he or she is aware of the nature of the document and is signing it freely and voluntarily.

Witness: _____   Witness: _____

Address: _____   Address: _____

Telephone: _____   Telephone: _____

STATE OF NEW HAMPSHIRE

COUNTY OF _____

The foregoing instrument was acknowledged before me this _____ day of _____, 19_____, by _____

Notary Public/Justice of the Peace _____

My Commission Expires: _____

Declaration

Declaration made this _____ day of _____ (month, year). I, _____, being of sound mind, willfully and voluntarily make known my desire that my dying shall not be artificially prolonged under the circumstances set forth below, do hereby declare:

If at any time I should have an incurable injury, disease, or illness certified to be a terminal condition or a permanently unconscious condition by 2 physicians who have personally examined me, one of whom shall be my attending physician, and the physicians have determined that my death will occur whether or not life-sustaining procedures are utilized or that I will remain in a permanently unconscious condition and where the application of life-sustaining procedures would serve only to artificially prolong the dying process, I direct that such procedures be withheld or withdrawn, and that I be permitted to die naturally with only the administration of medication, sustenance, or the performance of any medical procedure deemed necessary to provide me with comfort care. I realize that situations could arise in which the only way to allow me to die would be to discontinue artificial nutrition and hydration. In carrying out any instruction I have given under this section, I authorize that artificial nutrition and hydration not be started or, if started, be discontinued. (yes) (no) (Circle your choice and initial beneath it. If you do not choose "yes", artificial nutrition and hydration will be provided and will not be removed.)

In the absence of my ability to give directions regarding the use of such life-sustaining procedures, it is my intention that this declaration shall be honored by my family and physicians as the final expression of my right to refuse medical or surgical treatment and accept the consequences of such refusal.

I understand the full import of this declaration, and I am emotionally and mentally competent to make this declaration.

Signed _____

State of _____

County _____

We, the [declarant and] following witnesses, being duly sworn each declare to the notary public or justice of the peace of other official signing below as follows:

1. The declarant signed the instrument as a free and voluntary act for the purposes expressed, or expressly directed another to sign for him.

2. Each witness signed at the request of the declarant, in his presence, and in the presence of the other witness.

3. To the best of my knowledge, at the time of the signing the declarant was at least 18 years of age, and was of sane mind and under no constraint or undue influence.

Witness name _____ Witness name _____

Address _____ Address _____

Telephone _____ Telephone _____

New Hampshire

The affidavit shall be made before a notary public or justice of the peace of other official authorized to administer oaths in the place of execution, who shall not also serve as a witness, and who shall complete and sign a certificate in content and form substantially as follows:

Sworn to and signed before my by _____, declarant
_____ and _____, witnesses on
_____.

Signature _____

Official Capacity _____

Declaration of a Desire for a Natural Death

I, _____, being of sound mind, desire that, as specified below, my life not be prolonged by extraordinary means or by artificial nutrition or hydration if my condition is determined to be terminal and incurable or if I am diagnosed as being in a persistent vegetative state. I am aware and understand that this writing authorizes a physician to withhold or discontinue extraordinary means or artificial nutrition or hydration, in accordance with my specifications set forth below;

(Initial any of the following, as desired):

_____ If my condition is determined to be terminal and incurable, I authorize the following:

 _____ My physician may withhold or discontinue extraordinary means only.

 _____ In addition to withholding or discontinuing extraordinary means if such means are necessary, my physician may withhold or discontinue either artificial nutrition or hydration, or both.

_____ If my physician determines that I am in a persistent vegetative state, I authorize the following:

 _____ My physician may withhold or discontinue extraordinary means only.

 _____ In addition to withholding or discontinuing extraordinary means if such means are necessary, my physician may withhold or discontinue either artificial nutrition or hydration, or both.

This the _____ day of _____, 199_____.

Signature _____

I hereby state that the declarant, _____, being of sound mind signed the above declaration in my presence and that I am not related to the declarant by blood or marriage and that I do not know or have a reasonable expectation that I would be entitled to any portion of the estate of the declarant under any existing will or codicil of the declarant or as an heir under the Intestate Succession Act if the declarant died on this date without a will. I also state that I am not the declarant's attending physician or an employee of the declarant's attending physician, or an employee of a health facility in which the declarant is a patient or an employee of a nursing home or any group-care home where the declarant resides. I further state that I do not now have any claim against the declarant.

Witness (name) _____

(Address) _____

(Telephone) _____

Witness (name) _____

(Address) _____

(Telephone) _____

North Carolina

The clerk or the assistant clerk, or a notary public may, upon proper proof, certify the declaration as follows:

'Certificate'

I, _____, Clerk (Assistant Clerk) of Superior Court or Notary Public (circle one as appropriate) for _____ County hereby certify that _____, the declarant, appeared before me and swore to me and to the witnesses in my presence that this instrument is his Declaration Of A Desire For A Natural Death, and that he had willingly and voluntarily made and executed it as his free act and deed for the purposes expressed in it.

'I further certify that _____ and _____, witnesses, appeared before me and swore that they witnessed _____, declarant, sign the attached declaration, believing him to be of sound mind; and also swore that at the time they witnessed the declaration (i) they were not related within the third degree to the declarant or to the declarant's spouse, and (ii) they did not know or have a reasonable expectation that they would be entitled to any portion of the estate of the declarant upon the declarant's death under any will of the declarant or codicil thereto then existing or under the Intestate Succession Act as it provides at that time, and (iii) they were not a physician attending the declarant or an employee of an attending physician or an employee of a health facility in which the declarant was a patient or an employee of a nursing home or any group-care home in which the declarant resided, and (iv) they did not have a claim against the declarant. I further certify that I am satisfied as to the genuineness and due execution of the declaration.

'This the _____ day of _____, 199___.

Clerk (Assistant Clerk) of Superior Court or Notary Public (circle one as appropriate) for the County of

_____

Statutory Form Durable Power of Attorney for Health Care Warning to Person Executing This Document

This is an important legal document which is authorized by the general laws of this state. Before executing this document, you should know these important facts:

You must be at least eighteen years of age and a resident of the state of North Dakota for this document to be legally valid and binding.

This document gives the person you designate as your agent (the attorney in fact) the power to make health care decisions for you. Your agent must act consistently with your desires as stated in this document or otherwise made known.

Except as you otherwise specify in this document, this document gives your agent the power to consent to your doctor not giving treatment or stopping treatment necessary to keep you alive.

Notwithstanding this document, you have the right to make medical and other health care decisions for yourself so long as you can give informed consent with respect to the particular decision.

This document gives your agent authority to request, consent to, refuse to consent to, or to withdraw consent for any care, treatment, service, or procedure to maintain, diagnose, or treat a physical or mental condition if you are unable to do so yourself. This power is subject to any statement of your desires and any limitation that you include in this document. You may state in this document any types of treatment that you do not desire. In addition, a court can take away the power of your agent to make health care decisions for you if your agent authorizes anything that is illegal; acts contrary to your known desires; or where your desires are not known, does anything that is clearly contrary to your best interest.

Unless you specify a specific period, this power will exist until you revoke it. Your agent's power and authority ceases upon your death.

You have the right to revoke the authority of your agent by notifying your agent or your treating doctor, hospital, or other health care provider orally or in writing of the revocation.

Your agent has the right to examine your medical records and to consent to their disclosure unless you limit this right in this document.

This document revokes any prior durable power of attorney for health care.

You should carefully read and follow the witnessing procedure described at the end of this form. This document will not be valid unless you comply with the witnessing procedure.

If there is anything in this document that you do not understand, you should ask a lawyer to explain it to you.

Your agent may need this document immediately in case of an emergency that requires a decision concerning your health care. Either keep this document where it is immediately available to your agent and alternate agents, if any, or give each of them an executed copy of this document. You should give your doctor an executed copy of this document.

North Dakota

1. DESIGNATION OF HEALTH CARE AGENT. I, _____

_____

(insert your name and address)

do hereby designate and appoint: _____

_____

(insert name, address, and telephone number of one individual only as your agent to make health care decisions for you. None of the following may be designated as your agent: your treating health care provider, a nonrelative employee of your treating health care provider, an operator of a long-term care facility, or a nonrelative employee of an operator of a long-term care facility.) as my attorney in fact (agent) to make health care decisions for me as authorized in this document. For the purpose of this document, "health care decision" means consent, refusal of consent, or withdrawal of consent to any care, treatment, service, or procedure to maintain, diagnose, or treat an individual's physical or mental condition.

2. CREATION OF DURABLE POWER OF ATTORNEY FOR HEALTH CARE. By this document I intend to create a durable power of attorney for health care.

3. GENERAL STATEMENT OF AUTHORITY GRANTED. Subject to any limitations in this document, I hereby grant to my agent full power and authority to make health care decisions for me to the same extent that I could make such decisions for myself if I had the capacity to do so. In exercising this authority, my agent shall make health care decisions that are consistent with my desires as stated in this document or otherwise made known to my agent, including my desires concerning obtaining or refusing or withdrawing life-prolonging care, treatment, services, and procedures.

(If you want to limit the authority of your agent to make health care decisions for you, you can state the limitations in paragraph 4, "Statement of Desires, Special Provisions, and Limitations", below. You can indicate your desires by including a statement of your desires in the same paragraph.)

4. STATEMENT OF DESIRES, SPECIAL PROVISIONS, AND LIMITATIONS. (Your agent must make health care decisions that are consistent with your known desires. You can, but are not required to, state your desires in the space provided below. You should consider whether you want to include a statement of your desires concerning life-prolonging care, treatment, services, and procedures. You can also include a statement of your desires concerning other matters relating to your health care. You can also make your desires known to your agent by discussing your desires with your agent or by some other means. If there are any types of treatment that you do not want to be used, you should state them in the space below. If you want to limit in any other way the authority given your agent by this document, you should state the limits in the space below. If you do not state any limits, your agent will have broad powers to make health care decisions for you, except to the extent that there are limited provided by law.)

In exercising the authority under this durable power of attorney for health care, my agent shall act consistently with my desires as stated below and is subject to the special provisions and limitations stated below:

a. Statement of desires concerning life-prolonging care, treatment, services, and procedures:

_____

_____

_____

b. Additional statement of desires, special provisions, and limitations regarding health care decisions:

_____

_____

_____

(You may attach additional pages if you need more space to complete your statement. If you attach additional pages, you must date and sign EACH of the additional pages at the same time you date and sign this document.) If you wish to make a gift of any bodily organ you may do so pursuant to North Dakota Century Code chapter 23-06.2, the Uniform Anatomical Gift Act.

5. INSPECTION AND DISCLOSURE OF INFORMATION RELATING TO MY PHYSICAL OR MENTAL HEALTH. Subject to any limitations in this document, my agent has the power and authority to do all of the following:

a. Request, review, and receive any information, verbal or written, regarding my physical or mental health, including medical and hospital records.

b. Execute on my behalf any releases or other documents that may be required in order to obtain this information.

c. Consent to the disclosure of this information.

(If you want to limit the authority of your agent to receive and disclose information relating to your health, you must state the limitations in paragraph 4, "Statement of Desires, Special Provisions, and Limitations", above.)

6. SIGNING DOCUMENTS, WAIVERS, AND RELEASES. Where necessary to implement the health care decisions that my agent is authorized by this document to make, my agent has the power and authority to execute on my behalf all of the following:

a. Documents titled or purporting to be a "Refusal to Permit Treatment" and "Leaving Hospital Against Medical Advice".

b. Any necessary waiver or release from liability required by a hospital or physician.

7. DURATION. (Unless you specify a shorter period in the space below, this power of attorney will exist until it is revoked.)

This durable power of attorney for health care expires on

_____

(Fill in this space ONLY if you want the authority of your agent to end on a specific date.)

8. DESIGNATION OF ALTERNATE AGENTS. (You are not required to designate any alternate agents but you may do so. Any alternate agent you designate will be able to make the same health care decisions as the agent you designated in paragraph 1, above, in the event that agent is unable or ineligible to act as your agent. If the agent you designated is your spouse, he or she becomes ineligible to act as your agent if your marriage is dissolved. Your agent may withdraw whether or not you are capable of designating another agent.)

If the person designated as my agent in paragraph 1 is not available or becomes ineligible to act as my agent to make a health care decision for me or loses the mental capacity to make health care decisions for me, or if I revoke that person's appointment or authority to act as my agent to make health care decisions for me, then I designate and appoint the following persons to serve as my agent to make health care decisions for me as authorized in this document, such persons to serve in the order listed below:

a. First Alternate Agent: _____

_____

(Insert name, address, and telephone number of first alternate agent.)

North Dakota

b. Second Alternate Agent: _____

_____

(Insert name, address, and telephone number of second alternate agent.)

9. PRIOR DESIGNATIONS REVOKED. I revoke any prior durable power of attorney for health care.

DATE AND SIGNATURE OF PRINCIPAL
(YOU MUST DATE AND SIGN THIS POWER OF ATTORNEY)

I sign my name to this Statutory Form Durable Power of Attorney for Health Care on _____ (date) at _____ (city) _____ (state)

(you sign here) _____

(THIS POWER OF ATTORNEY WILL NOT BE VALID UNLESS IT IS SIGNED BY TWO (2) QUALIFIED WITNESSES WHO ARE PRESENT WHEN YOU SIGN OR ACKNOWLEDGE YOUR SIGNATURE. IF YOU HAVE ATTACHED ANY ADDITIONAL PAGES TO THIS FORM, YOU MUST DATE AND SIGN EACH OF THE ADDITIONAL PAGES AT THE SAME TIME YOU DATE AND SIGN THIS POWER OF ATTORNEY.)

STATEMENT OF WITNESSES

This document must be witnessed by two (2) qualified adult witnesses. None of the following may be used as a witness:

1. A person you designate as your agent or alternate agent;
2. A health care provider;
3. An employee of a health care provider;
4. The operator of a long-term care facility;
5. An employee of an operator of a long-term care facility;
6. Your spouse;
7. A person related to you by blood or adoption;
8. A person entitled to inherit any part of your estate upon your death; or
9. A person who has, at the time of executing this document, any claim against your estate.

I declare under penalty of perjury that the person who signed or acknowledged this document is personally known to me to be the principal, that the principal signed or acknowledged this durable power of attorney in my presence, that the principal appears to be of sound mind and under no duress, fraud, or undue influence, that I am not the person appointed as attorney in fact by this document, and that I am not a health care provider; an employee of a health care provider; the operator of a long-term care facility; an employee of an operator of a long-term care facility; the principal's spouse; a person related to the spouse by blood or adoption; a person entitled to inherit any part of the principal's estate upon death; nor a person who has, at the time of executing this document, any claim against the principal's estate.

Signature: _____ Residence Address: _____

Print Name: _____ _____

Date: _____ Telephone: _____

Signature: _____ Residence Address: _____

Print Name: _____ _____

Date: _____ Telephone: _____

10. ACCEPTANCE OF APPOINTMENT OF POWER OF ATTORNEY. I accept this appointment and agree to serve as agent for health care decisions. I understand I have a duty to act consistently with the desires of the principal as expressed in this appointment. I understand that this document gives me authority over health care decisions for the principal only if the principal becomes incapable. I understand that I must act in good faith in exercising my authority under this power of attorney. I understand that the principal may revoke this power of attorney at any time in any manner.

If I choose to withdraw during the time the principal is competent I must notify the principal of my decision. If I choose to withdraw when the principal is incapable of making the principal's health care decisions, I must notify the principal's physician.

(Signature of agent/date) _____

(Signature of alternate agent/date) _____

Declaration

Declaration made this _____ day of _____ (month, year).

I, _____, being at least eighteen years of age and of sound mind, willfully and voluntarily make known my desire that my life must not be artificially prolonged under the circumstances set forth below, and do hereby declare:

1. If at any time I should have an incurable condition caused by injury, disease, or illness certified to be a terminal condition by two physicians, and where the application of life-prolonging treatment would serve only to artificially prolong the process of my dying and my attending physician determines that my death is imminent whether or not life-prolonging treatment is utilized, I direct that such treatment be withheld or withdrawn, and that I be permitted to die naturally.

2. In the absence of my ability to give directions regarding the use of such life-prolonging treatment, it is my intention that this declaration by honored by my family and physicians as the final expression of my legal right to refuse medical or surgical treatment and accept the consequences of that refusal, which is death.

3. If I have been diagnosed as pregnant and that diagnosis is known to my physician, this declaration is not effective during the course of my pregnancy.

4. I understand the full import of this declaration, and I am emotionally and mentally competent to make this declaration.

5. I understand that I may revoke this declaration at any time.

Signed _____

City, County and State of Residence _____

The declarant has been personally known to me and I believe the declarant to be of sound mind. I am not related to the declarant by blood or marriage, nor would I be entitled to any portion of the declarant's estate upon the declarant's death. I am not the declarant's attending physician, a person who has a claim against any portion of the declarant's estate upon the declarant's death, or a person directly financially responsible for the declarant's medical care.

Witness (name) _____

(Address) _____

(Telephone) _____

Witness (name) _____

(Address) _____

(Telephone) _____

Notice to Adult Executing This Health Care Durable Power of Attorney

This is an important legal document. Before executing this document, you should know these facts:

This document gives the person you designate (the attorney in fact) the power to make MOST health care decisions for you if you lose the capacity to make informed health care decisions for yourself. This power is effective only when your attending physician determines that you have lost the capacity to make informed health care decisions for yourself and, notwithstanding this document, as long as you have the capacity to make informed health care decisions for yourself, you retain the right to make all medical and other health care decisions for yourself.

You may include specific limitations in this document on the authority of the attorney in fact to make health care decisions for you.

Subject to any specific limitations you include in this document, if your attending physician determines that you have lost the capacity to make an informed decision on a health care matter, the attorney in fact GENERALLY will be authorized by this document to make health care decisions for you to the same extent as you could make those decisions yourself, if you had the capacity to do so. The authority of the attorney in fact to make health care decisions for you GENERALLY will include the authority to give informed consent, to refuse to give informed consent, or to withdraw informed consent to any care, treatment, service, or procedure to maintain, diagnose, or treat a physical or mental condition.

HOWEVER, even if the attorney in fact has general authority to make health care decisions for you under this document, the attorney in fact NEVER will be authorized to do any of the following:

(1) Refuse or withdraw informed consent to life-sustaining treatment (unless your attending physician and one other physician who examines you determine, to a reasonable degree of medical certainty and in accordance with reasonable medical standards, that either of the following applies:

(a) You are suffering from an irreversible, incurable and untreatable condition caused by disease, illness or injury from which (i) there can be no recovery and (ii) your death is likely to occur within a relatively short time if life-sustaining treatment is not administered, and your attending physician additionally determines, to a reasonable degree of medical certainty and in accordance with reasonable medical standards, that there is no reasonable possibility that you will regain the capacity to make informed health care decisions for yourself.

(b) You are in a state of permanent unconsciousness that is characterized by you being irreversibly unaware of yourself and your environment and by a total loss of cerebral cortical functioning, resulting in you having no capacity to experience pain or suffering, and your attending physician additionally determines, to a reasonable degree of medical certainty and in accordance with reasonable medical standards, that there is no reasonable possibility that you will regain the capacity to make informed heath care decisions for yourself);

(2) Refuse or withdraw informed consent to health care necessary to provide you with comfort care (except that, if he is not prohibited from doing so under (4) below, the attorney in fact could refuse or withdraw informed consent to the provision of nutrition or hydration to you as described under (4) below. (YOU SHOULD UNDERSTAND THAT COMFORT CARE IS DEFINED IN OHIO LAW TO MEAN AR-

TIFICIALLY OR TECHNOLOGICALLY ADMINISTERED SUSTENANCE (NUTRITION) OR FLUIDS (HYDRATION) WHEN ADMINISTERED TO DIMINISH YOUR PAIN OR DISCOMFORT, NOT TO POSTPONE YOUR DEATH, AND ANY OTHER MEDICAL OR NURSING PROCEDURE, TREATMENT, INTERVENTION, OR OTHER MEASURE THAT WOULD BE TAKEN TO DIMINISH YOUR PAIN OR DISCOMFORT, NOT TO POSTPONE YOUR DEATH. CONSEQUENTLY, IF YOUR ATTENDING PHYSICIAN WERE TO DETERMINE THAT A PREVIOUSLY DESCRIBED MEDICAL OR NURSING PROCEDURE, TREATMENT, INTERVENTION, OR OTHER MEASURE WILL NOT OR NO LONGER WILL SERVE TO PROVIDE COMFORT TO YOU OR ALLEVIATE YOUR PAIN, THEN, SUBJECT TO (4) BELOW, YOUR ATTORNEY IN FACT WOULD BE AUTHORIZED TO REFUSE OR WITHDRAW INFORMED CONSENT TO THE PROCEDURE, TREATMENT, INTERVENTION, OR OTHER MEASURE.);

(3) Refuse or withdraw informed consent to health care for you if you are pregnant and if the refusal or withdrawal would terminate the pregnancy (unless the pregnancy or health care would pose a substantial risk to your life, or unless your attending physician and at least one other physician who examines you determine, to a reasonable degree of medical certainty and in accordance with reasonable medical standards, that the fetus would not be born alive);

(4) Refuse or withdraw informed consent to the provision of artificially or technologically administered sustenance (nutrition) or fluids (hydration) to you, unless

(a) you are in a terminal condition or in a permanently unconscious state.

(b) Your attending physician and at least one other physician who has examined you determine, to a reasonable degree of medical certainty and in accordance with reasonable medical standards, that nutrition or hydration will not or no longer will serve to provide comfort to you or alleviate your pain.

(c) if, but only if, you are in a permanently unconscious state, you authorize the attorney in fact to refuse or withdraw informed consent to the provision of nutrition or hydration to you by doing both of the following in this document:

(i) including a statement in capital letters that the attorney in fact may refuse or withdraw informed consent to the provision of nutrition or hydration to you if you are in a permanently unconscious state and if the determination that nutrition or hydration will not or no longer will serve to provide comfort to you or alleviate your pain is made, or checking or otherwise marking a box or line (if any) that is adjacent to a similar statement on this document;

(ii) placing your initial or signature underneath or adjacent to the statement, check or other mark previously described.

(d) Your attending physician determines, in good faith, that you authorized the attorney in fact to refuse or withdraw informed consent to the provision of nutrition or hydration to you if you are in a permanently unconscious state by complying with the requirements of (4)(c)(i) and (ii) above.

(5) Withdraw informed consent to any health care to which you previously consented, unless a change in your physical condition has significantly decreased the benefit of that health care to you, or unless the health care is not, or is no longer, significantly effective in achieving the purposes for which you consented to its use.

Additionally, when exercising his authority to make health care decisions for you, the attorney in fact will have to act consistently with your desires or, if your desires are unknown, to act in your best interest. You may express your desires to the attorney in fact by including them in this document or by making them known to him in another manner.

When acting pursuant to this document, the attorney in fact GENERALLY will have the same rights that you have to receive information about proposed health care, to review health care records, and to consent to the disclosure of health care records. You can limit that right in this document if you so choose.

Generally, you may designate any competent adult as the attorney in fact under this document. However, you cannot designate your attending physician or the administrator of any nursing home in which you are receiving care as the attorney in fact under this document. Additionally, you cannot designate an employee or agent of your attending physician or an employee or agent of a health care facility at which you are being treated as the attorney in fact under this document, unless either type of employee or agent is a competent adult and related to you by blood, marriage, or adoption, or unless either type of employee or agent is a competent adult and you and the employee or agent are members of the same religious order.

This document has no expiration date under Ohio law, but you may choose to specify a date upon which your durable power of attorney for health care generally will expire. However, if you specify an expiration date and then lack the capacity to make informed health care decisions for yourself on that date, the document and the power it grants to your attorney in fact will continue in effect until you regain the capacity to make informed health care decisions for yourself.

You have the right to revoke the designation of the attorney in fact and the right to revoke this entire document at any time and in any manner. Any such revocation generally will be effective when you express your intention to make the revocation. However, if you made your attending physician aware of this document, any such revocation will be effective only when you communicate it to your attending physician, or when a witness to the revocation or other health care personnel to whom the revocation is communicated by such a witness communicates it to your physician.

If you execute this document and create a valid durable power of attorney for health care with it, it will revoke any prior, valid durable power of attorney for health care that you created, unless you indicate otherwise in this document.

This document is not valid as a durable power of attorney for health care unless it is acknowledged before a notary public or is signed by at least two adult witnesses who are present when you sign or acknowledge your signature. No person who is related to you by blood, marriage, or adoption may be a witness. The attorney in fact, your attending physician, and the administrator of any nursing home in which you are receiving care also are ineligible to be witnesses.

If there is anything in this document that you do not understand, you should ask your lawyer to explain it to you.

I have read this notice and I understand it. I want my attorney in fact to have the powers described in my Durable Power of Attorney for Health-Care Decisions, even if those are broader than described in this notice.

Name _____

Date _____

Statement Regarding "Terminal Condition" and "Permanently Unconscious State"

I make this statement to satisfy the requirements of Ohio Revised Code Annotated § 2133.02 (A)(2), and I intend it to be treated as part of my Declaration.

I intend that my Declaration be implemented if I am in either a "TERMINAL CONDITION" or a "PERMANENTLY UNCONSCIOUS STATE," and in any other condition I have initialed in my "Supplement to Directive or Declaration to Physicians," at "3. These are the Judgments I want my physician to consider in making treatment decisions," attached to my Declaration.

By "TERMINAL CONDITION," I MEAN ANY DISEASE, INJURY OR OTHER CONDITION FROM WHICH THERE CAN BE NO RECOVERY, AND THAT IN REASONABLE MEDICAL JUDGMENT PROBABLY WILL RESULT IN MY DEATH SOON IF LIFE-SUSTAINING TREATMENT IS NOT USED.

By "PERMANENTLY UNCONSCIOUS STATE," I MEAN ANY CONDITION OF IRREVERSIBLE UNCONSCIOUSNESS IN WHICH, BASED ON REASONABLE MEDICAL STANDARDS, I AM UNAWARE OF MY SELF OR MY ENVIRONMENT, THERE IS TOTAL OR NEAR-TOTAL LOSS OF CEREBRAL CORTICAL FUNCTIONING, AND FROM WHICH RECOVERY OF CONSCIOUSNESS TO THE EXTENT OF BEING ABLE TO THINK AND COMMUNICATE IS UNLIKELY.

Advance Directive for Health Care

I, _____, being of sound mind and eighteen (18) years of age or older, willfully and voluntarily make known my desire, by my instructions to others through my living will, or by my appointment of a health care proxy, or both, that my life shall not be artificially prolonged under the circumstances set forth below. I thus do hereby declare:

I. Living Will

a. If my attending physician and another physician determine that I am no longer able to make decisions regarding my medical treatment, I direct my attending physician and other health care providers, pursuant to the Oklahoma Rights of the Terminally Ill or Persistently Unconscious Act, to withhold or withdraw treatment from me under the circumstances I have indicated below by my signature. I understand that I will be given treatment that is necessary for my comfort or to alleviate my pain.

b. If I have a terminal condition:

(1) I direct that life-sustaining treatment shall be withheld or withdrawn if such treatment would only prolong my process of dying, and if my attending physician and another physician determine that I have an incurable and irreversible condition that even with the administration of life-sustaining treatment will cause my death within six (6) months.

(signature) _____

(2) I understand that the subject of the artificial administration of nutrition and hydration (food and water) that will only prolong the process of dying from an incurable and irreversible condition is of particular importance. I understand that if I do not sign this paragraph, artificially administered nutrition and hydration will be administered to me. I further understand that if I sign this paragraph, I am authorizing the withholding or withdrawal of artificially administered nutrition (food) and hydration (water).

(signature) _____

(3) I direct that (add other medical directives, if any)

_____

_____

(signature) _____

c. If I am persistently unconscious:

(1) I direct that life-sustaining treatment be withheld or withdrawn if such treatment will only serve to maintain me in an irreversible condition, as determined by my attending physician and another physician, in which thought and awareness of self and environment are absent.

(signature) _____

(2) I understand that the subject of the artificial administration of nutrition and hydration (food and water) for individuals who have become persistently unconscious is of particular importance. I understand

that if I do not sign this paragraph, artificially administered nutrition and hydration will be administered to me. I further understand that if I sign this paragraph, I am authorizing the withholding or withdrawal of artificially administered nutrition (food) and hydration (water).

(3) I direct that (add other medical directives, if any)

_____

_____

(signature) _____

II. My Appointment of My Health Care Proxy

a. If my attending physician and another physician determine that I am no longer able to make decisions regarding my medical treatment, I direct my attending physician and other health care providers pursuant to the Oklahoma Rights of the Terminally Ill or Persistently Unconscious Act to follow the instruction of _____, whom I appoint as my health care proxy. If my health care proxy is unable or unwilling to serve, I appoint _____ as my alternate health care proxy with the same authority. My health care proxy is authorized to make whatever medical treatment decision I could make if I were able, except that decisions regarding life-sustaining treatment can be made by my health care proxy or alternate health care proxy only as I indicate in the following sections.

b. If I have a terminal condition:

(1) I authorize my health care proxy to direct that life-sustaining treatment be withheld or withdrawn if such treatment would only prolong my process of dying and if my attending physician and another physician determine that I have an incurable and irreversible condition that even with the administration of life-sustaining treatment will cause my death within six (6) months.

(signature) _____

(2) I understand that the subject of the artificial administration of nutrition and hydration (food and water) is of particular importance. I understand that if I do not sign this paragraph, artificially administered nutrition (food) or hydration (water) will be administered to me. I further understand that if I sign this paragraph, I am authorizing the withholding or withdrawal of artificially administered nutrition and hydration.

(signature) _____

(3) I authorize my health care proxy to (add other medical directives, if any)

_____

_____

(signature) _____

c. If I am persistently unconscious:

(1) I authorize my health care proxy to direct that life-sustaining treatment be withheld or withdrawn if such treatment will only serve to maintain me in an irreversible condition, as determined by my attending physician and another physician, in which thought and awareness of self and environment are absent.

(signature) _____

(2) I understand that the subject of the artificial administration of nutrition and hydration (food and water) is of particular importance. I understand that if I do not sign this paragraph, artificially administered

nutrition (food) and hydration (water) will be administered to me. I further understand that if I sign this paragraph, I am authorizing the withholding and withdrawal of artificially administered nutrition and hydration.

(signature) _____

(3) I authorize my health care proxy to (add other medical directives, if any)

_____

_____

(signature) _____

III. Conflicting Provision

I understand that if I have completed both a living will and have appointed a health care proxy, and if there is a conflict between my health care proxy's decision and my living will, I want my power of attorney to take precedence.

(signature) _____

IV. Other Provisions

a. I understand that if I have been diagnosed as pregnant and that diagnosis is known to my attending physician, this advance directive shall have no force or effect during the course of my pregnancy.

b. In the absence of my ability to give directions regarding the use of life-sustaining procedures, it is my intention that this advance directive shall be honored by my family and physicians as the final expression of my legal right to refuse medical or surgical treatment including, but not limited to, the administration of any life-sustaining procedures, and I accept the consequences of such refusal.

c. This advance directive shall be in effect until it is revoked.

d. I understand that I may revoke this advance directive at any time.

e. I understand and agree that if I have any prior directives, and if I sign this advance directive, my prior directives are revoked.

f. I understand the full importance of this advance directive and I am emotionally and mentally competent to make this advance directive.

Signed this _____ day of _____, 19_____

(Signature) _____

City, County and State of Residence _____

This advance directive was signed in my presence.

(Signature of Witness) _____

(Address/telephone) _____

(Signature of Witness) _____

(Address/telephone) _____

Power of Attorney for Health Care

I appoint _____, whose address is _____,
and whose telephone number is _____, as my attorney-in-fact for health care decisions.
I appoint _____, whose address is _____,
and whose telephone number is _____, as my alternative attorney-in-fact for health
care decisions. I authorize my attorney-in-fact appointed by this document to make health care decisions for
me when I am incapable of making my own health care decisions. I have read the warning below and
understand the consequences of appointing a power of attorney for health care.

I direct that my attorney-in-fact comply with the following instructions or limitations: _____

_____

In addition, I direct that my attorney-in-fact have authority to make decisions regarding the following:

—Withholding or withdrawal of life-sustaining procedures with the understanding that death may
result.

—Withholding or withdrawal of artificially administered hydration or nutrition or both with the
understanding that dehydration, malnutrition and death may result.

(Signature of person making appointment/date) _____

WARNING TO PERSON APPOINTING A POWER OF ATTORNEY FOR HEALTH CARE

This is an important legal document. It creates a power of attorney for health care. Before signing this
document, you should know these important facts:

This document gives the person you designate as your attorney-in-fact the power to make health care
decisions for you, subject to any limitations, specifications or statement of your desires that you include in
this document.

For this document to be effective, your attorney-in-fact must accept the appointment in writing.

The person you designate in this document has a duty to act consistently with your desires as stated in
this document or otherwise made known or, if your desires are unknown, to act in a manner consistent with
what the person in good faith believes to be in your best interest. The person you designate in this document
does, however, have the right to withdraw from this duty at any time.

This power will continue in effect for a period of seven years unless you become unable to participate in
health care decisions for yourself during that period. If this occurs, the power will continue in effect until
you are able to participate in those decisions again.

You have the right to revoke the appointment of the person designated in this document at any time by
notifying that person or your health care provider of the revocation orally or in writing.

Despite this document, you have the right to make medical and other health care decisions for yourself
as long as you are able to participate knowledgeably in those decisions.

If there is anything in this document that you do not understand, you should ask a lawyer to explain it to
you. This power of attorney will not be valid for making health care decisions unless it is signed by two
qualified witnesses who are personally known to you and who are present when you sign or acknowledge
your signature.

Oregon

DECLARATION OF WITNESSES

We declare that the principal is personally known to us, that the principal signed or acknowledged the principal's signature on this power of attorney for health care in our presence, that the principal appears to be of sound mind and not under duress, fraud or undue influence, that neither of us is the person appointed as attorney-in-fact by this document or the principal's attending physician. Witnessed By:

(Signature of Witness/Date) _____

(Printed Name of Witness) _____

(Address/Telephone) _____

(Signature of Witness/Date) _____

(Printed Name of Witness) _____

(Address/Telephone) _____

ACCEPTANCE OF APPOINTMENT OF POWER OF ATTORNEY

I accept this appointment and agree to serve as attorney-in-fact for health care decisions. I understand I have a duty to act consistently with the desires of the principal as expressed in this appointment. I understand that this document gives me authority over health care decisions for the principal only if the principal becomes incapable. I understand that I must act in good faith in exercising my authority under this power of attorney. I understand that the principal may revoke this power of attorney at any time in any manner, and that I have a duty to inform the principal's attending physician promptly upon any revocation.

(Signature of Attorney-in-fact/Date) _____

(Printed Name) _____

(Signature of Alternate Attorney-in-fact/Date) _____

(Printed Name) _____

Directive to Physicians

Directive made this _____ day of _____ (month, year). I
_____, being of sound mind, willfully and voluntarily make known my
desire that my life shall not be artificially prolonged under the circumstances set forth below and do hereby
declare:

1. If at any time I should have an incurable injury, disease or illness certified to be a terminal condition
by two physicians, one of whom is the attending physician, and where the application of life-sustaining
procedures would serve only to artificially prolong the moment of my death and where my physician
determines that my death is imminent whether or not life-sustaining procedures are utilized, I direct that
such procedures be withheld or withdrawn, and that I be permitted to die naturally.

2. In the absence of my ability to give directions regarding the use of such life-sustaining procedures, it
is my intention that this directive shall be honored by my family and physician(s) as the final expression of
my legal right to refuse medical or surgical treatment and accept the consequences from such refusal.

3. I understand the full import of this directive and I am emotionally and mentally competent to make
this directive.

Signed _____

City, County and State of Residence _____

I hereby witness this directive and attest that:

(1) I personally know the Declarant and believe the Declarant to be of sound mind.

(2) To the best of my knowledge, at the time of the execution of this directive, I:

(a) Am not related to the Declarant by blood or marriage.

(b) Do not have any claim on the estate of the Declarant.

(c) Am not entitled to any portion of the Declarant's estate by any will or by operation of law, and

(d) Am not a physician attending the Declarant, a person employed by a physician attending the
Declarant or a person employed by a health facility in which the Declarant is a patient.

(3) I understand that if I have not witnessed this directive in good faith I may be responsible for any
damages that arise out of giving this directive its intended effect.

Witness _____

Address _____

Telephone _____

Witness _____

Address _____

Telephone _____

PENNSYLVANIA _____

Declaration

I, _____, being of sound mind, willfully and voluntarily make this declaration to be followed if I become incompetent. This declaration reflects my firm and settled commitment to refuse life-sustaining treatment under the circumstances indicated below.

I direct my attending physician to withhold or withdraw life-sustaining treatment that serves only to prolong the process of my dying, if I should be in a terminal condition or in a state of permanent unconsciousness.

I direct that treatment be limited to measures to keep me comfortable and to relieve pain, including any pain that might occur by withholding or withdrawing life-sustaining treatment.

In addition, if I am in the condition described above, I feel especially strong about the following forms of treatment:

I (   ) do (   ) do not want cardiac resuscitation.

I (   ) do (   ) do not want mechanical respiration.

I (   ) do (   ) do not want tube feeding or any other artificial or invasive form of nutrition (food) or hydration (water).

I (   ) do (   ) do not want blood or blood products.

I (   ) do (   ) do not want any form of surgery or invasive diagnostic tests.

I (   ) do (   ) do not want kidney dialysis.

I (   ) do (   ) do not want antibiotics.

I realize that if I do not specifically indicate my preference regarding any of the forms of treatment listed above, I may receive that form of treatment.

Other instructions:

I (   ) do (   ) do not want to designate another person as my surrogate to make medical treatment decisions for me if I should be incompetent and in a terminal condition or in a state of permanent unconsciousness. Name and address of surrogate (if applicable):

Name and address of substitute surrogate (if surrogate designated above is unable to serve):

I made this declaration on the _____ day of _____ (month, year).

Declarant's signature: _____

Declarant's address: _____

The declarant or the person on behalf of and at the direction of the declarant knowingly and voluntarily signed this writing by signature or mark in my presence.

Witness's signature: _____

Witness's address: _____

Witness's telephone: _____

Witness's signature: _____

Witness's address: _____

Witness's telephone: _____

Statutory Form Durable Power of Attorney for Health Care

WARNING TO PERSON EXECUTING THIS DOCUMENT

This is an important legal document which is authorized by the general laws of this state. Before executing this document, you should know these important facts:

You must be at least eighteen (18) years of age and a resident of the state of Rhode Island for this document to be legally valid and binding.

This document gives the person you designate as your agent (the attorney in fact) the power to make health care decisions for you. Your agent must act consistently with your desires as stated in this document or otherwise made known.

Except as you otherwise specify in this document, this document gives your agent the power to consent to your doctor not giving treatment or stopping treatment necessary to keep you alive.

Notwithstanding this document, you have the right to make medical and other health care decisions for yourself so long as you can give informed consent with respect to the particular decision. In addition, no treatment may be given to you over your objection at the time, and health care necessary to keep you alive may not be stopped or withheld if you object at the time.

This document gives your agent authority to consent, to refuse to consent or to withdraw consent to any care, treatment, service, or procedure to maintain, diagnose or treat a physical or mental condition. This power is subject to any statement of your desires and any limitation that you include in this document. You may state in this document any types of treatment that you do not desire. In addition, a court can take away the power of your agent to make health care decisions for you if your agent:

(1) Authorized anything that is illegal,

(2) Acts contrary to your known desires, or

(3) Where your desires are not known, does anything that is clearly contrary to your best interests.

Unless you specify a specific period, this power will exist until you revoke it. Your agent's power and authority ceases upon your death.

You have the right to revoke the authority of your agent by notifying your agent or your treating doctor, hospital, or other health care provider orally or in writing of the revocation.

Your agent has the right to examine your medical records and to consent to their disclosure unless you limit this right in this document.

This document revokes any prior durable power of attorney for health care.

You should carefully read and follow the witnessing procedure described at the end of this form. This document will not be valid unless you comply with the witnessing procedure.

If there is anything in this document that you do not understand, you should ask a lawyer to explain it to you.

Your agent may need this document immediately in case of an emergency that requires a decision concerning your health care. Either keep this document where it is immediately available to your agent and alternate agents or give each of them an executed copy of this document. You may also want to give your doctor an executed copy of this document.

Rhode Island

(1) DESIGNATION OF HEALTH CARE AGENT. I, _____

_____

_____

(insert your name and address) _____

do hereby designate and appoint: _____

(insert name, address, and telephone number of one individual only as your agent to make health care decisions for you. None of the following may be designated as your agent: (1) your treating health care provider, (2) a nonrelative employee of your treating health care provider, (3) an operator of a community care facility, or (4) a nonrelative employee of an operator of a community care facility.) as my attorney in fact (agent) to make health care decisions for me as authorized in this document. For the purposes of this document, "health care decision" means consent, refusal of consent, or withdrawal of consent to any care, treatment, service, or procedure to maintain, diagnose, or treat an individual's physical or mental condition.

(2) CREATION OF DURABLE POWER OF ATTORNEY FOR HEALTH CARE. By this document I intend to create a durable power of attorney for health care.

(3) GENERAL STATEMENT OF AUTHORITY GRANTED. Subject to any limitations in this document, I hereby grant to my agent full power and authority to make health care decisions for me to the same extent that I could make such decisions for myself if I had the capacity to do so. In exercising this authority, my agent shall make health care decisions that are consistent with my desires as stated in this document or otherwise made known to my agent, including, but not limited to, my desires concerning obtaining or refusing or withdrawing life-prolonging care, treatment, services, and procedures.

(If you want to limit the authority of your agent to make health care decisions for you, you can state the limitations in paragraph 4 ("Statement of Desires, Special Provisions, and Limitations") below. You can indicate your desires by including a statement of your desires in the same paragraph.)

(4) STATEMENT OF DESIRES, SPECIAL PROVISIONS AND LIMITATIONS. (Your agent must make health care decisions that are consistent with your known desires. You can, but are not required to, state your desires in the space provided below. You should consider whether you want to include a statement of your desires concerning life-prolonging care, treatment, services, and procedures. You can also include a statement of your desires concerning other matters relating to your health care. You can also make your desires known to your agent by discussing your desires with your agent or by some other means. If there are any types of treatment that you do not want to be used, you should state them in the space below. If you want to limit in any other way the authority given your agent by this document, you should state the limits in the space below. If you do not state any limits, your agent will have broad powers to make health care decisions for you, except to the extent that there are limits provided by law.)

In exercising the authority under this durable power of attorney for health care, my agent shall act consistently with my desires as stated below and is subject to the special provisions and limitations stated below:

(a) Statement of desires concerning life-prolonging care, treatment, services, and procedures:

_____

_____

_____

_____

_____

_____

_____

(b) Additional statement of desires, special provisions, and limitations regarding health care decisions:

_____

_____

_____

_____

_____

_____

_____

_____

(You may attach additional pages if you need more space to complete your statement. If you attach additional pages, you must date and sign EACH of the additional pages at the same time you date and sign this document.) If you wish to make a gift of any bodily organ you may do so pursuant to the Uniform Anatomical Gift Act.

(5) INSPECTION AND DISCLOSURE OF INFORMATION RELATING TO MY PHYSICAL OR MENTAL HEALTH. Subject to any limitations in this document, my agent has the power and authority to do all of the following:

(a) Request, review, and receive any information, verbal or written, regarding my physical or mental health, including, but not limited to, medical and hospital records.

(b) Execute on my behalf any releases or other documents that may be required in order to obtain this information.

(c) Consent to disclosure of this information

(If you want to limit the authority of your agent to receive and disclose information relating to your health, you must state the limitations in paragraph 4 ("Statement of desires, special provisions, and limitations") above.)

(6) SIGNING DOCUMENTS, WAIVERS AND RELEASES. Where necessary to implement the health care decisions that my agent is authorized by this document to make, my agent has the power and authority to execute on my behalf all of the following:

(a) Documents titled or purporting to be a "Refusal to Permit Treatment" and "Leaving Hospital Against Medical Advice."

(b) Any necessary waiver or release from liability required by a hospital or physician.

(7) DURATION. (Unless you specify a shorter period in the space below, this power of attorney will exist until it is revoked.)

This durable power of attorney for health care expires on _____. (Fill in this space ONLY if you want the authority of your agent to end on a specific date.)

(8) DESIGNATION OF ALTERNATE AGENTS.

(You are not required to designate any alternate agents but you may do so. Any alternate agent you designate will be able to make the same health care decisions as the agent you designated in paragraph 1, above, in the event that agent is unable or ineligible to act as your agent. If the agent you designated is your spouse, he or she becomes ineligible to act as your agent if your marriage is dissolved.)

Rhode Island

If the person designated as my agent in paragraph 1 is not available or becomes ineligible to act as my agent to make a health care decision for me or loses the mental capacity to make health care decisions for me, or if I revoke that person's appointment or authority to act as my agent to make health care decisions for me, then I designate and appoint the following persons to serve as my agent to make health care decisions for me as authorized in this document, such persons to serve in the order listed below:

    (A) First Alternate Agent: _____
(Insert name, address, and telephone number of first alternate agent.)
    (B) Second Alternate Agent: _____
(Insert name, address, and telephone number of second alternate agent.)
    (9) PRIOR DESIGNATIONS REVOKED. I revoke any prior durable power of attorney for health care.

DATE AND SIGNATURE OF PRINCIPAL
(YOU MUST DATE AND SIGN THIS POWER OF ATTORNEY)

    I sign my name to this Statutory Form Durable Power of Attorney for Health Care on _____
(Date) at _____ (City) _____ (State)

(You sign here) _____

(THIS POWER OF ATTORNEY WILL NOT BE VALID UNLESS IT IS SIGNED BY TWO (2) QUALIFIED WITNESSES WHO ARE PRESENT WHEN YOU SIGN OR ACKNOWLEDGE YOUR SIGNATURE. IF YOU HAVE ATTACHED ANY ADDITIONAL PAGES TO THIS FORM, YOU MUST DATE AND SIGN EACH OF THE ADDITIONAL PAGES AT THE SAME TIME YOU DATE AND SIGN THIS POWER OF ATTORNEY.)

STATEMENT OF WITNESSES

(This document must be witnessed by two (2) qualified adult witnesses. None of the following may be used as a witness:

    (1) A person you designated as your agent or alternate agent,
    (2) A health care provider,
    (3) An employee of a health care provider,
    (4) The operator of a community care facility,
    (5) An employee of an operator of a community care facility.

    At least one of the witnesses must make the additional declaration set out following the place where the witnesses sign.)

    I declare under penalty of perjury that the person who signed or acknowledged this document is personally known to me to be the principal, that the principal signed or acknowledged this durable power of attorney in my presence, that the principal appears to be of sound mind and under no duress, fraud or undue influence, that I am not the person appointed as attorney in fact by this document, and that I am not a health care provider, an employee of a health care provider, the operator of a community care facility, nor an employee of an operator of a community care facility.

Signature: _____   Residence Address: _____

Print Name: _____   _____

Date: _____   Telephone: _____

Signature: _____   Residence Address: _____

Print Name: _____   _____

Date: _____   Telephone: _____

(AT LEAST ONE OF THE ABOVE WITNESSES MUST ALSO SIGN THE FOLLOWING DECLARATION.)

I further declare under penalty of perjury that I am not related to the principal by blood, marriage, or adoption, and, to the best of my knowledge, I am not entitled to any part of the estate of the principal upon the death of the principal under a will now existing or by operation of law.

Signature: _____

Print Name: _____

Signature: _____

Print Name: _____

Declaration

I, _____, being of sound mind willfully and voluntarily make known my desire that my dying shall not be artificially prolonged under the circumstances set forth below, do hereby declare:

If I should have an incurable or irreversible condition that will cause my death within a relatively short time, and if I am unable to make decisions regarding my medical treatment, I direct my attending physician to withhold or withdraw procedures that merely prolong the dying process and are not necessary to my comfort, or to alleviate pain.

This authorization includes ( ) does not include ( ) the withholding or withdrawal of artificial feeding (check only one box above.)

Signed this _____ day of _____, _____.

Signature _____

Address _____

The declarant is personally known to me and voluntarily signed this document in my presence.

Witness _____

Address _____

Telephone _____

Witness _____

Address _____

Telephone _____

Power of Attorney

INFORMATION ABOUT THIS DOCUMENT

THIS IS AN IMPORTANT LEGAL DOCUMENT. BEFORE SIGNING THIS DOCUMENT, YOU SHOULD KNOW THESE IMPORTANT FACTS:

1. THIS DOCUMENT GIVES THE PERSON YOU NAME AS YOUR AGENT THE POWER TO MAKE HEALTH CARE DECISIONS FOR YOU IF YOU CANNOT MAKE THE DECISION FOR YOURSELF. THIS POWER INCLUDES THE POWER TO MAKE DECISIONS ABOUT LIFE-SUSTAINING TREATMENT. UNLESS YOU STATE OTHERWISE, YOUR AGENT WILL HAVE THE SAME AUTHORITY TO MAKE DECISIONS ABOUT YOUR HEALTH CARE AS YOU WOULD HAVE.

2. THIS POWER IS SUBJECT TO ANY LIMITATIONS OR STATEMENTS OF YOUR DESIRES THAT YOU INCLUDE IN THIS DOCUMENT. YOU MAY STATE IN THIS DOCUMENT ANY TREATMENT YOU DO NOT DESIRE OR TREATMENT YOU WANT TO BE SURE YOU RECEIVE. YOUR AGENT WILL BE OBLIGATED TO FOLLOW YOUR INSTRUCTIONS WHEN MAKING DECISIONS ON YOUR BEHALF. YOU MAY ATTACH ADDITIONAL PAGES IF YOU NEED MORE SPACE TO COMPLETE THE STATEMENT.

3. AFTER YOU HAVE SIGNED THIS DOCUMENT, YOU HAVE THE RIGHT TO MAKE HEALTH CARE DECISIONS FOR YOURSELF IF YOU ARE MENTALLY COMPETENT TO DO SO. AFTER YOU HAVE SIGNED THIS DOCUMENT, NO TREATMENT MAY BE GIVEN TO YOU OR STOPPED OVER YOUR OBJECTION IF YOU ARE MENTALLY COMPETENT TO MAKE THAT DECISION.

4. YOU HAVE THE RIGHT TO REVOKE THIS DOCUMENT, AND TERMINATE YOUR AGENT'S AUTHORITY, BY INFORMING EITHER YOUR AGENT OR YOUR HEALTH CARE PROVIDER ORALLY OR IN WRITING.

5. IF THERE IS ANYTHING IN THIS DOCUMENT THAT YOU DO NOT UNDERSTAND, YOU SHOULD ASK A SOCIAL WORKER, LAWYER, OR OTHER PERSON TO EXPLAIN IT TO YOU.

6. THIS POWER OF ATTORNEY WILL NOT BE VALID UNLESS TWO PERSONS SIGN AS WITNESSES. EACH OF THESE PERSONS MUST EITHER WITNESS YOUR SIGNING OF THE POWER OF ATTORNEY OR WITNESS YOUR ACKNOWLEDGMENT THAT THE SIGNATURE ON THE POWER OF ATTORNEY IS YOURS.

THE FOLLOWING PERSONS MAY NOT ACT AS WITNESSES:

A. YOUR SPOUSE; YOUR CHILDREN, GRANDCHILDREN, AND OTHER LINEAL DESCENDANTS; YOUR PARENTS, GRANDPARENTS, AND OTHER LINEAL ANCESTORS; YOUR SIBLINGS AND THEIR LINEAL DESCENDANTS; OR A SPOUSE OF ANY OF THESE PERSONS.

B. A PERSON WHO IS DIRECTLY FINANCIALLY RESPONSIBLE FOR YOUR MEDICAL CARE.

C. A PERSON WHO IS NAMED IN YOUR WILL, OR, IF YOU HAVE NO WILL, WHO WOULD INHERIT YOUR PROPERTY BY INTESTATE SUCCESSION.

D. A BENEFICIARY OF A LIFE INSURANCE POLICY ON YOUR LIFE.

E. THE PERSONS NAMED IN THE HEALTH CARE POWER OF ATTORNEY AS YOUR AGENT OR SUCCESSOR AGENT.

F. YOUR PHYSICIAN OR AN EMPLOYEE OF YOUR PHYSICIAN.

G. ANY PERSON WHO WOULD HAVE A CLAIM AGAINST ANY PORTION OF YOUR ESTATE (PERSONS TO WHOM YOU OWE MONEY).

IF YOU ARE A PATIENT IN A HEALTH FACILITY, NO MORE THAN ONE WITNESS MAY BE AN EMPLOYEE OF THAT FACILITY.

7. YOUR AGENT MUST BE A PERSON WHO IS 18 YEARS OLD OR OLDER AND OF SOUND MIND. IT MAY NOT BE YOUR DOCTOR OR ANY OTHER HEALTH CARE PROVIDER THAT IS NOW PROVIDING YOU WITH TREATMENT; OR AN EMPLOYEE OF YOUR DOCTOR OR PROVIDER; OR A SPOUSE OF THE DOCTOR, PROVIDER, OR EMPLOYEE; UNLESS THE PERSON IS A RELATIVE OF YOURS.

8. YOU SHOULD INFORM THE PERSON THAT YOU WANT HIM OR HER TO BE YOUR HEALTH CARE AGENT. YOU SHOULD DISCUSS THIS DOCUMENT WITH YOUR AGENT AND YOUR PHYSICIAN AND GIVE EACH A SIGNED COPY. IF YOU ARE IN A HEALTH CARE FACILITY OR A NURSING CARE FACILITY, A COPY OF THIS DOCUMENT SHOULD BE INCLUDED IN YOUR MEDICAL RECORD.

HEALTH CARE POWER OF ATTORNEY

(S.C. STATUTORY FORM)

1. DESIGNATION OF HEALTH CARE AGENT

I, _____ (Principal), hereby appoint:

(Agent) _____

(Address) _____

_____

Home Telephone: _____

Work Telephone: _____

as my agent to make health care decision for me as authorized in this document.

2. EFFECTIVE DATE AND DURABILITY

By this document I intend to create a durable power of attorney effective upon, and only during, any period of mental incompetence.

3. AGENT'S POWERS

I grant to my agent full authority to make decisions for me regarding my health care. In exercising this authority, my agent shall follow my desires as stated in this document or otherwise expressed by me or known to my agent. In making any decision, my agent shall attempt to discuss the proposed decision with me to determine my desires if I am able to communicate in any way. If my agent cannot determine the choice I would want made, then my agent shall make a choice for me based upon what my agent believes to be in my best interests. My agent's authority to interpret my desires is intended to be as broad as possible, except for any limitations I may state below.

Accordingly, unless specifically limited by Section E, below, my agent is authorized as follows:

A. To consent, refuse, or withdraw consent to any and all types of medical care, treatment, surgical procedures, diagnostic procedures, medication, and the use of mechanical or other procedures that affect any bodily function, including, but not limited to, artificial respiration, nutritional support and hydration, and cardiopulmonary resuscitation;

B. To authorize, or refuse to authorize, any medication or procedure intended to relieve pain, even though such use may lead to physical damage, addiction, or hasten the moment of, but not intentionally cause, my death;

C. To authorize my admission to or discharge, even against medical advice, from any hospital, nursing care facility, or similar facility or service;

D. To take any other action necessary to making, documenting, and assuring implementation of decisions concerning my health care, including, but not limited to, granting any waiver or release from liability required by any hospital, physician, nursing care provider, or other health care provider; signing any documents relating to refusals of treatment or the leaving of a facility against medical advice, and pursuing any legal action in my name, and at the expense of my estate to force compliance with my wishes as determined by my agent, or to seek actual or punitive damages for the failure to comply.

E. The powers granted above do not include the following powers or are subject to the following rules or limitations:

_____

_____

_____

4. ORGAN DONATION (INITIAL ONLY ONE)
My agent may _____; may not _____ consent to the donation of all or any of my tissues or organs for purposes of transplantation.

5. EFFECT ON DECLARATION OF A DESIRE FOR A NATURAL DEATH (LIVING WILL)
I understand that if I have a valid Declaration of a Desire for a Natural Death, the instructions contained in the Declaration will be given effect in any situation to which they are applicable. My agent will have authority to make decisions concerning my health care only in situations to which the Declaration does not apply.

6. STATEMENT OF DESIRES AND SPECIAL PROVISIONS
With respect to any Life-Sustaining Treatment, I direct the following:
(INITIAL ONLY ONE OF THE FOLLOWING 4 PARAGRAPHS)
(1) _____ GRANT OF DISCRETION TO AGENT. I do not want my life to be prolonged nor do I want life-sustaining treatment to be provided or continued if my agent believes the burdens of the treatment outweigh the expected benefits. I want my agent to consider the relief of suffering, my personal beliefs, the expense involved and the quality as well as the possible extension of my life in making decisions concerning life-sustaining treatment.
OR
(2) _____ DIRECTIVE TO WITHHOLD OR WITHDRAW TREATMENT. I do not want my life to be prolonged and I do not want life-sustaining treatment:
a. if I have a condition that is incurable or irreversible and, without the administration of life-sustaining procedures, expected to result in death within a relatively short period of time; or
b. if I am in a state of permanent unconsciousness.
OR
(3) _____ DIRECTIVE FOR MAXIMUM TREATMENT. I want my life to be prolonged to the greatest extent possible, within the standards of accepted medical practice, without regard to my condition, the chances I have for recovery, or the cost of the procedures.
OR
(4) _____ DIRECTIVE IN MY OWN WORDS:

_____

_____

_____

7. STATEMENT OF DESIRES REGARDING TUBE FEEDING
With respect to Nutrition and Hydration provided by means of a nasogastric tube or tube into the stomach, intestines, or veins, I wish to make clear that (INITIAL ONLY ONE)

_____ I do not want to receive these forms of artificial nutrition and hydration, and they may be withhold or withdrawn under the conditions given above.

OR

_____ I do want to receive these forms of artificial nutrition and hydration.

IF YOU DO NOT INITIAL EITHER OF THE ABOVE STATEMENTS, YOUR AGENT WILL NOT HAVE AUTHORITY TO DIRECT THAT NUTRITION AND HYDRATION NECESSARY FOR COMFORT CARE OR ALLEVIATION OF PAIN BE WITHDRAWN.

8. SUCCESSORS

If an agent named by me dies, becomes legally disabled, resigns, refuses to act, becomes unavailable, or if an agent who is my spouse is divorced or separated from me, I name the following as successors to my agent, each to act alone and successively, in the order named.

A. First Alternate Agent: _____

Address: _____

Telephone: _____

B. Second Alternate Agent: _____

Address: _____

Telephone: _____

9. ADMINISTRATIVE PROVISIONS

A. I revoke any prior Health Care Power of Attorney and any provisions relating to health care of any other prior power of attorney.

B. This power of attorney is intended to be valid in any jurisdiction in which it is presented.

10. UNAVAILABILITY OF AGENT

If at any relevant time the Agent or Successor Agents named herein are unable or unwilling to make decision concerning my health care, and those decisions are to be made by a guardian, by the Probate Court, or by a surrogate pursuant to the Adult Health Care Consent Act, it is my intention that the guardian, Probate Court, or surrogate make those decisions in accordance with my directions as stated in this document.

BY SIGNING HERE I INDICATE THAT I UNDERSTAND THE CONTENTS OF THIS DOCUMENT AND THE EFFECT OF THIS GRANT OF POWERS TO MY AGENT.

I sign my name to this Health Care Power of Attorney on the _____ day of _____, 19 _____. My current home address is:

_____

_____

Signature: _____

Name: _____

WITNESS STATEMENT

I declare, on the basis of information and belief, that the person who signed or acknowledged this document (the principal) is personally known to me, that he/she signed or acknowledged this Health Care Power of Attorney in my presence, and that he/she appears to be of sound mind and under no duress, fraud, or undue influence. I am not related to the principal by blood, marriage, or adoption, either as a spouse, a lineal ancestor, descendant of the parents of the principal, or spouse of any of them. I am not directly financially responsible for the principal's medical care. I am not entitled to any portion of the principal's estate upon his decease, whether under any will or as an heir by intestate succession, nor am I the beneficiary of an insurance policy on the principal's life, nor do I have a claim against the principal's estate as of this time. I am not the principal's attending physician, nor an employee of the attending physician. No more than one witness is an employee of a health facility in which the principal is a patient. I am not appointed as Health Care Agent or Successor Health Care Agent by this document.

Witness No. 1

Signature: _____

Print Name: _____

Residence Address: _____

Telephone: _____

Date: _____

Witness No. 2

Signature: _____

Print Name: _____

Residence Address: _____

Telephone: _____

Date: _____

STATE OF SOUTH CAROLINA

COUNTY OF _____

DECLARATION OF A DESIRE FOR A NATURAL DEATH

I, _____, Declarant, being at least eighteen years of age and a resident of and domiciled in the City of _____, County of _____, State of South Carolina, make this declaration this _____ day of _____, 19 _____.

I wilfully and voluntarily make known my desire that no life-sustaining procedures be used to prolong my dying if my condition is terminal or if I am in a state of permanent unconsciousness, and I declare:

If at any time I have a condition certified to be a terminal condition by two physicians who have personally examined me, one of whom is my attending physician, and the physicians have determined that my death could occur within a reasonably short period of time without the use of life-sustaining procedures or if the physicians certify that I am in a state of permanent unconsciousness and where the application of life-sustaining procedures would serve only to prolong the dying process, I direct that the procedures be withheld or withdrawn, and that I be permitted to die naturally with only the administration of medication or the performance of any medical procedure necessary to provide me with comfort care.

INSTRUCTIONS CONCERNING ARTIFICIAL NUTRITION AND HYDRATION

INITIAL ONE OF THE FOLLOWING STATEMENTS

If my condition is terminal and could result in death within a reasonably short time,

_____ I direct that nutrition and hydration BE PROVIDED through any medically indicated means, including medically or surgically implanted tubes.

_____ I direct that nutrition and hydration NOT BE PROVIDED through any medically indicated means, including medically or surgically implanted tubes.

South Carolina

INITIAL ONE OF THE FOLLOWING STATEMENTS

If I am in a persistent vegetative state or other condition of permanent unconsciousness,

_____ I direct that nutrition and hydration BE PROVIDED through any medically indicated means, including medically or surgically implanted tubes.

_____ I direct that nutrition and hydration NOT BE PROVIDED through any medically indicated means, including medically or surgically implanted tubes.

In the absence of my ability to give directions regarding the use of life-sustaining procedures, it is my intention that this Declaration be honored by my family and physicians and any health facility in which I may be a patient as the final expression of my legal right to refuse medical or surgical treatment, and I accept the consequences from the refusal.

I am aware that this Declaration authorizes a physician to withhold or withdraw life-sustaining procedures. I am emotionally and mentally competent to make this Declaration.

APPOINTMENT OF AN AGENT (OPTIONAL)

1. You may give another person authority to revoke this declaration on your behalf. If you wish to do so, please enter that person's name in the space below.

Name of Agent with Power to Revoke: _____

Address: _____

Telephone Number: _____

2. You may give another person authority to enforce this declaration on your behalf. If you wish to do so, please enter that person's name in the space below.

Name of Agent with Power to Enforce: _____

Address: _____

Telephone Number: _____

REVOCATION PROCEDURES

THIS DECLARATION MAY BE REVOKED BY ANY ONE OF THE FOLLOWING METHODS. HOWEVER, A REVOCATION IS NOT EFFECTIVE UNTIL IT IS COMMUNICATED TO THE ATTENDING PHYSICIAN.

(1) BY BEING DEFACED, TORN, OBLITERATED, OR OTHERWISE DESTROYED, IN EXPRESSION OF YOUR INTENT TO REVOKE, BY YOU OR BY SOME PERSON IN YOUR PRESENCE AND BY YOUR DIRECTION. REVOCATION BY DESTRUCTION OF ONE OR MORE OF MULTIPLE ORIGINAL DECLARATIONS REVOKES ALL OF THE ORIGINAL DECLARATION;

(2) BY A WRITTEN REVOCATION SIGNED AND DATED BY YOU EXPRESSING YOUR INTENT TO REVOKE;

(3) BY YOUR ORAL EXPRESSION OF YOUR INTENT TO REVOKE THE DECLARATION. AN ORAL REVOCATION COMMUNICATED TO THE ATTENDING PHYSICIAN BY A PERSON OTHER THAN YOU IS EFFECTIVE ONLY IF:

(a) THE PERSON WAS PRESENT WHEN THE ORAL REVOCATION WAS MADE;

(b) THE REVOCATION WAS COMMUNICATED TO THE PHYSICIAN WITHIN A REASONABLE TIME.

(c) YOUR PHYSICAL OR MENTAL CONDITION MAKES IT IMPOSSIBLE FOR THE PHYSICIAN TO CONFIRM THROUGH SUBSEQUENT CONVERSATION WITH YOU THAT THE REVOCATION HAS OCCURRED.

TO BE EFFECTIVE AS A REVOCATION, THE ORAL EXPRESSION CLEARLY MUST INDICATE YOUR DESIRE THAT THE DECLARATION NOT BE GIVEN EFFECT OR THAT LIFE-SUSTAINING PROCEDURES BE ADMINISTERED;

(4) IF YOU, IN THE SPACE ABOVE, HAVE AUTHORIZED AN AGENT TO REVOKE THE DECLARATION, THE AGENT MAY REVOKE ORALLY OR BY A WRITTEN, SIGNED, AND DATED INSTRUMENT. AN AGENT MAY REVOKE ONLY IF YOU ARE INCOMPETENT TO DO SO. AN AGENT MAY REVOKE THE DECLARATION PERMANENTLY OR TEMPORARILY.

(5) BY YOUR EXECUTING ANOTHER DECLARATION AT A LATER TIME.

Signature of Declarant: _____

STATE OF _____ AFFIDAVIT

COUNTY OF _____

We, _____ and _____, the undersigned witnesses to the foregoing Declaration, dated the _____ day of _____, 19 _____, at least one of us being first duly sworn, declare to the undersigned authority, on the basis of our best information and belief, that the Declaration was on that date signed by the declarant as and for his DECLARATION OF A DESIRE FOR A NATURAL DEATH in our presence and we, at his request and in his presence, and in the presence of each other, subscribe our names as witnesses on that date. The declarant is personally known to us, and we believe him to be of sound mind. Each of us affirms that he is qualified as a witness to this Declaration under the provisions of the South Carolina Death With Dignity Act in that he is not related to the declarant by blood, marriage, or adoption, either as a spouse, lineal ancestor, descendant of the parents of the declarant, or spouse of any of them; nor directly financially responsible for the declarant's medical care; nor entitled to any portion of the declarant's estate upon his decease, whether under any will or as an heir by intestate succession; nor the beneficiary of a life insurance policy of the declarant; nor the declarant's attending physician; nor an employee of the attending physician; nor a person who has a claim against the declarant's decedent's estate as of this time. No more than one of us is an employee of a health facility in which the declarant is a patient. If the declarant is a resident in a hospital or nursing care facility at the date of execution of this Declaration, at least one of us is an ombudsman designated by the State Ombudsman, Office of the Governor.

Witness _____

Address/Telephone _____

Witness _____

Address/Telephone _____

Subscribed before me by _____, the declarant, and subscribed and sworn to before me by _____, the witness, this _____ day of _____, 19 _____.

Signature _____

Notary Public for _____

My commission expires: _____

SEAL

Living Will Declaration

This is an important legal document. This document directs the medical treatment you are to receive in the event you are unable to participate in your own medical decisions and you are in a terminal condition. This document may state what kind of treatment you want or do not want to receive.

This document can control whether you live or die. Prepare this document carefully. If you use this form, read it completely. You may want to seek professional help to make sure the form does what you intend and is completed without mistakes.

This document will remain valid and in effect until and unless you revoke it. Review this document periodically to make sure it continues to reflect your wishes. You may amend or revoke this document at any time by notifying your physician and other health-care providers. You should give copies of this document to your physician and your family. This form is entirely optional. If you choose to use this form, please note that the form provides signature lines for you, the two witnesses whom you have selected and a notary public.

TO MY FAMILY, PHYSICIANS, AND ALL THOSE CONCERNED WITH MY CARE:

I, _____, willfully and voluntarily make this declaration as a directive to be followed if I am in a terminal condition and become unable to participate in decisions regarding my medical care.

With respect to any life-sustaining treatment, I direct the following:

(Initial only one of the following optional directives if you agree. If you do not agree with any of the following directive, space is provided below for you to write your own directives.)

_____ NO LIFE-SUSTAINING TREATMENT. I direct that no life-sustaining treatment be provided. If life-sustaining treatment is begun, terminate it.

_____ TREATMENT FOR RESTORATION. Provide life-sustaining treatment only if and for so long as you believe treatment offers a reasonable possibility of restoring to me the ability to think and act for myself.

_____ TREAT UNLESS PERMANENTLY UNCONSCIOUS. If you believe that I am permanently unconscious and are satisfied that this condition is irreversible, then do not provide me with life-sustaining treatment, and if life-sustaining treatment is being provided to me, terminate it. If and so long as you believe that treatment has a reasonable possibility of restoring consciousness to me, then provide life-sustaining treatment.

_____ MAXIMUM TREATMENT. Preserve my life as long as possible, but do not provide treatment that is not in accordance with accepted medical standards as then in effect.

(Artificial nutrition and hydration is food and water provided by means of a nasogastric tube or tubes inserted into the stomach, intestines, or veins. If you do not wish to receive this form of treatment, you must initial the statement below which reads: "I intend to include this treatment, among the 'life-sustaining treatment' that may be withheld or withdrawn.")

With respect to artificial nutrition and hydration, I wish to make clear that

(Initial one only)

_____ I intend to include this treatment among the "life-sustaining treatment" that may be withheld or withdrawn.

_____ I do not intend to include this treatment among the "life-sustaining treatment" that may be withheld or withdrawn.

South Dakota

(If you do not agree with any of the printed directives and want to write your own, or if you want to write directives in addition to the printed provision, or if you want to express some of your other thoughts, you can do so here.)

_____

_____

_____

_____

_____

_____

Date: _____

Your signature: _____

Your address: _____

Type or print your signature: _____

The declarant voluntarily signed this document in my presence.

Witness: _____

Address: _____

Telephone: _____

Witness: _____

Address: _____

Telephone: _____

On this the _____ day of _____, _____, the declarant, _____, and witnesses, _____, and _____ personally appeared before the undersigned officer and signed the foregoing instrument in my presence. Dated this _____ day of _____, _____.

Notary Public _____

My commission expires: _____

Health Care Power of Attorney

WARNING TO PERSON EXECUTING THIS DOCUMENT

This is an important legal document. Before executing this document you should know these important facts.

This document gives the person you designate as your agent (the attorney in fact) the power to make health care decisions for you. Your agent must act consistently with your desires as stated in this document.

Except as you otherwise specify in this document, this document gives your agent the power to consent to your doctor not giving treatment or stopping treatment necessary to keep you alive.

Notwithstanding this document, you have the right to make medical and other health care decisions for yourself so long as you can give informed consent with respect to the particular decision. In addition, no treatment may be given to you over your objection, and health care necessary to keep you alive may not be stopped or withheld if you object at the time.

This document gives your agent authority to consent, to refuse to consent, or to withdraw consent to any care, treatment, service, or procedure to maintain, diagnose or treat a physical or mental condition. This power is subject to any limitations that you include in this document. You may state in this document any types of treatment that you do not desire. In addition, a court can take away the power of your agent to make health care decisions for you if your agent: (1) authorizes anything that is illegal; or (2) acts contrary to your desires as stated in this document.

You have the right to revoke the authority of your agent by notifying your agent or your treating physician, hospital or other health care provider orally or in writing of the revocation.

Your agent has the right to examine your medical records and to consent to their disclosure unless you limit this right in this document.

Unless you otherwise specify in this document, this document gives your agent the power after you die to: (1) authorize an autopsy; (2) donate your body or parts thereof for transplant or therapeutic or educational or scientific purposes; and (3) direct the disposition of your remains.

If there is anything in this document that you do not understand, you should ask an attorney to explain it to you.

I have read this warning and I understand it.

Signature _____

Date _____

Living Will

I, _____, willfully and voluntarily make known my desire that my dying shall not be artificially prolonged under the circumstances set forth below, and do hereby declare:

If at any time I should have a terminal condition and my attending physician has determined there is no reasonable medical expectation of recovery and which, as a medical probability, will result in my death, regardless of the use or discontinuance of medical treatment implemented for the purpose of sustaining life, or the life process, I direct that medical care be withheld or withdrawn, and that I be permitted to die naturally with only the administration of medications or the performance of any medical procedure deemed necessary to provide me with comfortable care or to alleviate pain.

ARTIFICIALLY PROVIDED NOURISHMENT AND FLUIDS:

By checking the appropriate line below, I specifically:

_____ Authorize the withholding or withdrawal of artificially provided food, water or other nourishment or fluids.

_____ DO NOT authorize the withholding or withdrawal of artificially provided food, water or other nourishment or fluids.

ORGAN DONOR CERTIFICATION:

Notwithstanding my previous declaration relative to the withholding or withdrawal of life-prolonging procedures, if as indicated below I have expressed my desire to donate my organs and/or tissues for transplantation, or any of them specifically designated herein, I do direct my attending physician, if I have been determined dead according to Tennessee Code Annotated, § 68-3-501(b), to maintain me on artificial support systems only for the period of time required to maintain the viability of and to remove such organs and/or tissues.

By checking the appropriate line below, I specifically:

_____ Desire to donate my organs and/or tissues for transplantation.

_____ Desire to donate my _____

(Insert specific organs and/or tissues for transplantation)

_____ DO NOT desire to donate my organs or tissues for transplantation.

In the absence of my ability to give directions regarding my medical care, it is my intention that this declaration shall be honored by my family and physician as the final expression of my legal right to refuse medical care and accept the consequences of such refusal.

The definitions of terms used herein shall be as set forth in the Tennessee Right to Natural Death Act, Tennessee Code Annotated, §32-11-103.

I understand the full import of this declaration, and I am emotionally and mentally competent to make this declaration.

In acknowledgment whereof, I do hereinafter affix my signature on this the _____ day of _____, 19_____.

Declarant _____

Tennessee

We, the subscribing witnesses hereto, are personally acquainted with and subscribe our names hereto at the request of the declarant, an adult, whom we believe to be of sound mind, fully aware of the action taken herein and its possible consequence.

We, the undersigned witnesses, further declare that we are not related to the declarant by blood or marriage; that we are not entitled to any portion of the estate of the declarant upon the declarant's decease under any will or codicil thereto presently existing or by operation of law then existing; that we are not the attending physician, an employee of the attending physician or a health facility in which the declarant is a patient; and that we are not persons who, at the present time, have a claim against any portion of the estate of the declarant upon the declarant's death.

Witness (name, address, telephone) _____

_____

Witness (name, address, telephone) _____

_____

STATE OF TENNESSEE

COUNTY OF _____

Subscribed, sworn to and acknowledged before me by _____, the declarant, and subscribed and sworn to before me by _____ and _____ _____, witnesses, this _____ day of _____, 19 _____.

Notary Public _____

My Commission Expires: _____

Information Concerning the Durable Power of Attorney for Health Care

THIS IS AN IMPORTANT LEGAL DOCUMENT. BEFORE SIGNING THIS DOCUMENT, YOU SHOULD KNOW THESE IMPORTANT FACTS:

Except to the extent you state otherwise, this document gives the person you name as your agent the authority to make any and all health care decisions for you in accordance with your wishes, including your religious and moral beliefs, when you are no longer capable of making them yourself. Because "health care" means any treatment, service, or procedure to maintain, diagnose, or treat your physical or mental condition, your agent has the power to make a broad range of health care decisions for you. Your agent may consent, refuse to consent, or withdraw consent to medical treatment and may make decisions about withdrawing or withholding life-sustaining treatment. Your agent may not consent to voluntary inpatient mental health services, convulsive treatment, psychosurgery, or abortion. A physician must comply with your agent's instructions or allow you to be transferred to another physician.

Your agent's authority begins when your doctor certifies that you lack the capacity to make health care decisions.

Your agent is obligated to follow your instructions when making decisions on your behalf. Unless you state otherwise, your agent has the same authority to make decisions about your health care as you would have had.

It is important that you discuss this document with your physician or other health care provider before you sign it to make sure that you understand the nature and range of decisions that may be made on your behalf. If you do not have a physician, you should talk with someone else who is knowledgeable about these issues and can answer your questions. You do not need a lawyer's assistance to complete this document, but if there is anything in this document that you do not understand, you should ask a lawyer to explain it to you.

The person you appoint as agent should be someone you know and trust. The person must be 18 years of age or older or a person under 18 years of age who has had the disabilities of minority removed. If you appoint your health or residential care provider (e.g., your physician or an employee of a home health agency, hospital, nursing home, or residential care home, other than a relative), that person has to choose between acting as your agent or as your health or residential care provider; the law does not permit a person to do both at the same time.

You should inform the person you appoint that you want the person to be your health care agent. You should discuss this document with your agent and your physician and give each a signed copy. You should indicate on the document itself the people and institutions who have signed copies. Your agent is not liable for health care decisions made in good faith on your behalf.

Even after you have signed this document, you have the right to make health care decisions for yourself as long as you are able to do so and treatment cannot be given to you or stopped over your objection. You have the right to revoke the authority granted to your agent by informing your agent or your health or residential care provider orally or in writing, or by your execution of a subsequent durable power of attorney for health care. Unless you state otherwise, your appointment of a spouse dissolves on divorce.

Texas

This document may not be changed or modified. If you want to make changes in the document, you must make an entirely new one.

You may wish to designate an alternate agent in the event that your agent is unwilling, unable or ineligible to act as your agent. Any alternate agent you designate has the same authority to make health care decisions for you.

THIS POWER OF ATTORNEY IS NOT VALID UNLESS IT IS SIGNED IN THE PRESENCE OF TWO OR MORE QUALIFIED WITNESSES. THE FOLLOWING PERSONS MAY NOT ACT AS WITNESSES:

    (1) the person you have designated as your agent;

    (2) your health or residential care provider or an employee of your health or residential care provider;

    (3) your spouse;

    (4) your lawful heirs or beneficiaries named in your will or a deed; or

    (5) creditor or persons who have a claim against you.

I have read the preceding statement, and I understand it.

Signature: _____

DURABLE POWER OF ATTORNEY FOR HEALTH CARE DESIGNATION OF HEALTH CARE AGENT.

    I, _____ (insert your name) appoint:

Name: _____

Address: _____

Phone: _____

as my agent to make any and all health care decisions for me, except to the extent I state otherwise in this document. This durable power of attorney for health care takes effect if I become unable to make my own health care decisions and this fact is certified in writing by my physician.

LIMITATIONS ON THE DECISION MAKING AUTHORITY OF MY AGENT ARE AS FOLLOWS:

_____

_____

DESIGNATION OF ALTERNATE AGENT.

    (You are not required to designate an alternate agent but you may do so. An alternate agent may make the same health care decisions as the designated agent if the designated agent is unable or unwilling to act as your agent. If the agent designated is your spouse, the designation is automatically revoked by law if your marriage is dissolved.)

    If the person designated as my agent is unable or unwilling to make health care decisions for me, I designate the following persons to serve as my agent to make health care decisions for me as authorized by this document, who serve in the following order:

A. First Alternate Agent

Name: _____

Address: _____

Phone: _____

B. Second Alternate Agent

Name: _____

Address: _____

Phone: _____

The original of this document is kept at _____
The following individuals or institutions have signed copies:

Name: _____

Address: _____

Name: _____

Address: _____

DURATION:

I understand that this power of attorney exists indefinitely from the date I execute this document unless I establish a shorter time or revoke the power of attorney. If I am unable to make health care decisions for myself when this power of attorney expires, the authority I have granted my agent continues to exist until the time I become able to make health care decisions for myself.

(IF APPLICABLE) This power of attorney ends on the following date: _____
PRIOR DESIGNATIONS REVOKED.

I revoke any prior durable power of attorney for health care.
ACKNOWLEDGMENT OF DISCLOSURE STATEMENT.

I have been provided with a disclosure statement explaining the effect of this document. I have read and understand that information contained in the disclosure statement.

Further statement of intentions: _____

_____

(YOU MUST DATE AND SIGN THIS POWER OF ATTORNEY)

I sign my name to this durable power of attorney for health care on _____ day of
_____ 19_____ at

(City and State) _____

(Signature) _____

(Print Name) _____

STATEMENT OF WITNESSES.

I declare under penalty of perjury that the principal has identified himself or herself to me, that the principal signed or acknowledged this durable power of attorney in my presence, that I believe the principal to be of sound mind, that the principal has affirmed that the principal is aware of the nature of the document and is signing it voluntarily and free from duress, that the principal requested that I serve as witness to the principal's execution of this document, that I am not the person appointed as agent by this document, and that I am not a provider of health or residential care, an employee of a provider of health or residential care, the operator of a community care facility, or an employee of an operator of a health care facility.

Texas

I declare that I am not related to the principal by blood, marriage, or adoption and that to the best of my knowledge I am not entitled to any part of the estate of the principal on the death of the principal under a will or by operation of law.

Witness Signature: _____

Print Name: _____

Date: _____

Address: _____

Witness Signature: _____

Print Name: _____

Date: _____

Address: _____

Directive to Physicians

Directive made this _____ day of _____ (month, year).

I _____, being of sound mind, wilfully and voluntarily make known my desire that my life shall not be artificially prolonged under the circumstances set forth in this directive.

1. If at any time I should have an incurable condition caused by injury, disease, or illness certified to be a terminal condition by two physicians, and if the application of life-sustaining procedures would serve only to artificially postpone the moment of my death, and if my attending physician determines that my death is imminent whether or not life-sustaining procedures are used, I direct that those procedures be withheld or withdrawn, and that I be permitted to die naturally.

2. In the absence of my ability to give directions regarding the use of those life-sustaining procedures, it is my intention that this directive be honored by my family and physicians as the final expression of my legal right to refuse medical or surgical treatment and accept the consequences from that refusal.

3. If I have been diagnosed as pregnant and that diagnosis is known to my physician, this directive has no effect during my pregnancy.

4. This directive is in effect until it is revoked.

5. I understand the full import of this directive and I am emotionally and mentally competent to make this directive.

6. I understand that I may revoke this directive at any time.

Signed _____

(City, County and State of Residence) _____

The declarant has been personally known to me and I believe the declarant to be of sound mind. I am not related to the declarant by blood or marriage. I would not be entitled to any portion of the declarant's estate on the declarant's death. I am not the attending physician of the declarant or an employee of the attending physician or a health facility in which the declarant is a patient. I am not a patient in the health care facility in which the declarant is a patient. I have no claim against any portion of the declarant's estate on the declarant's death.

Witness _____

Address _____

Telephone _____

Witness _____

Address _____

Telephone _____

U T A H _____

Special Power of Attorney

I, _____, of _____, this _____ day of _____, 199__, being of sound mind, wilfully and voluntarily appoint (name) _____ of (city) _____ as my agent and attorney-in-fact, without substitution, with lawful authority to execute a directive on my behalf under Section 75-2-1105, governing the care and treatment to be administered to or withheld from me at any time after I incur an injury, disease, or illness which renders me unable to give current directions to attending physicians and other providers of medical services.

I understand that "life-sustaining procedures" do not include the administration of medication or sustenance, or the performance of any medical procedure deemed necessary to provide comfort care, or to alleviate pain, unless my attorney-in-fact specifies these procedures be considered life-sustaining.

I have carefully selected my above-named agent with confidence in the belief that this person's familiarity with my desires, beliefs,and attitudes will result in directions to attending physicians and providers of medical services which would probably be the same as I would give if able to do so.

This power of attorney shall be and remain in effect from the time my attending physician certifies that I have incurred a physical or mental condition rendering me unable to give current directions to attending physicians or other providers of medical services as to my care and treatment.

Statement of my intentions: _____

_____

_____

Signature of Principal _____

STATE OF _____)
                               : ss.
County of _____)

On the _____ day of _____, _____, personally appeared before me _____, who duly acknowledged to me that he has read and fully understands the foregoing power of attorney, executed the same of his own volition and for the purposes set forth, and that he was acting under no constraint or undue influence whatsoever.

Notary Public _____

My commission expires: _____

Residing at: _____

_____

Directive to Physicians and Providers of Medical Services

(Pursuant to Section 75-2-1104, UCA)

This directive is made this _____ day of _____, _____.

1. I, _____, being of sound mind, willfully and voluntarily make known my desire that my life not be artificially prolonged by life-sustaining procedures except as I may otherwise provide in this directive.

2. I declare that if at any time I should have an injury, disease, or illness, which is certified in writing to be a terminal condition by two physicians who have personally examined me, and in the opinion of those physicians the application of life-sustaining procedures would serve only to unnaturally prolong the moment of my death and to unnaturally postpone or prolong the dying process, I direct that these procedure be withheld or withdrawn and my death be permitted to occur naturally.

3. I expressly intend this directive to be a final expression of my legal right to refuse medical or surgical treatment and to accept the consequences from this refusal which shall remain in effect notwithstanding my future inability to give current medical directions to treating physicians and other providers of medical services.

4. I understand that the term "life-sustaining procedure" does not include the administration of medication or sustenance, or the performance of any medical procedure deemed necessary to provide comfort care, or to alleviate pain, except to the extent I specify below that any of these procedures be considered life-sustaining.

5. I reserve the right to give current medical directions to physicians and other providers of medical services so long as I am able, even though these directions may conflict with the above written directive that life-sustaining procedures be withheld or withdrawn.

6. I understand the full import of this directive and declare that I am emotionally and mentally competent to make this directive.

Declarant's Signature _____

City, County and State of Residence _____

We witnesses certify that each of us is 18 years of age or older and each personally witnessed the declarant sign or direct the signing of this directive; that we are acquainted with the declarant and believe him to be of sound mind; that the declarant's desires are as expressed above; that neither of us is a person who signed the above directive on behalf of the declarant; that we are not related to the declarant by blood or marriage nor are we entitled to any portion of the declarant's estate according to the laws of intestate succession of this state or under any will or codicil of declarant; that we are not directly financially responsible for declarant's medical care; and that we are not agents of any health care facility in which the declarant may be a patient at the time of signing this directive.

Signature of Witness _____   Signature of Witness _____

Address _____   Address _____

Telephone _____   Telephone _____

Durable Power of Attorney for Health Care

INFORMATION CONCERNING THE DURABLE POWER OF ATTORNEY FOR HEALTH CARE

THIS IS AN IMPORTANT LEGAL DOCUMENT. BEFORE SIGNING THIS DOCUMENT, YOU SHOULD KNOW THESE IMPORTANT FACTS:

Except to the extent you state otherwise, this document gives the person you name as your agent the authority to make any and all health care decisions for you when you are no longer capable of making them yourself. "Health care" means any treatment, service or procedure to maintain, diagnose or treat your physical or mental condition. Your agent therefore can have the power to make a broad range of health care decisions for you. Your agent may consent, refuse to consent, or withdraw consent to medical treatment and may make decisions about withdrawing or withholding life-sustaining treatment.

You may state in this document any treatment you do not desire or treatment you want to be sure you receive. Your agent's authority will begin when your doctor certifies that you lack the capacity to make health care decisions. You may attach additional pages if you need more space to complete your statement.

Your agent will be obligated to follow your instructions when making decisions on your behalf. Unless you state otherwise, your agent will have the same authority to make decisions about your health care as you would have had.

It is important that you discuss this document with your physician or other health care providers before you sign it to make sure that you understand the nature and range of decisions which may be made on your behalf. If you do not have a physician, you should talk with someone else who is knowledgeable about these issues and can answer your questions. You do not need a lawyer's assistance to complete this document, but if there is anything in this document that you do not understand, you should ask a lawyer to explain it to you.

The person you appoint as agent should be someone you know and trust and must be at least 18 years old. If you appoint your health or residential care provider (e.g. your physician, or an employee of a home health agency, hospital, nursing home, or residential care home, other than a relative), that person will have to choose between acting as your agent or as your health or residential care provider; the law does not permit a person to do both at the same time.

You should inform the person you appoint that you want him or her to be your health care agent. You should discuss this document with your agent and your physician and give each a signed copy. You should indicate on the document itself the people and institutions who will have signed copies. Your agent will not be liable for health care decisions made in good faith on your behalf.

Even after you have signed this document, you have the right to make health care decisions for yourself as long as you are able to do so, and treatment cannot be given to you or stopped over your objection. You have the right to revoke the authority granted to your agent by informing him or her or your health care provider orally or in writing.

THIS DOCUMENT MAY NOT BE CHANGED OR MODIFIED. IF YOU WANT TO MAKE CHANGES IN THE DOCUMENT YOU MUST MAKE AN ENTIRELY NEW ONE.

You may wish to designate an alternate agent in the event that your agent is unwilling, unable or

Vermont

ineligible to act as your agent. Any alternate agent you designate will have the same authority to make health care decisions for you.

THIS POWER OF ATTORNEY WILL NOT BE VALID UNLESS IT IS SIGNED IN THE PRESENCE OF TWO (2) OR MORE QUALIFIED WITNESSES WHO MUST BOTH BE PRESENT WHEN YOU SIGN OR ACKNOWLEDGE YOUR SIGNATURE. THE FOLLOWING PERSONS MAY NOT ACT AS WITNESSES:

—the person you designated as your agent;

—your health or residential care provider or one of their employees;

—your spouse;

—your lawful heirs or beneficiaries named in your will or a deed;

—creditors or persons who have a claim against you.

I have read this statement and I understand it.

Signature _____

DURABLE POWER OF ATTORNEY FOR HEALTH CARE

I, _____, hereby appoint _____ of _____ as my agent to make any and all health care decisions for me, except to the extent I state otherwise in this document. This durable power of attorney for health care shall take effect in the event I become unable to make my own health care decisions.

(a) STATEMENT OF DESIRES, SPECIAL PROVISIONS, AND LIMITATIONS REGARDING HEALTH CARE DECISIONS.

Here you may include any specific desires or limitations you deem appropriate, such as when or what life-sustaining measures should be withheld; directions whether to continue or discontinue artificial nutrition and hydration; or instructions to refuse any specific types of treatment that are inconsistent with your religious beliefs or unacceptable to you for any other reason.

_____

_____

_____

_____

_____

(attach additional pages as necessary)

(b) THE SUBJECT OF LIFE-SUSTAINING TREATMENT IS OF PARTICULAR IMPORTANCE. For your convenience in dealing with that subject, some general statements concerning the withholding or removal or life-sustaining treatment are set forth below. IF YOU AGREE WITH ONE OF THESE STATEMENTS, YOU MAY INCLUDE THE STATEMENT IN THE BLANK SPACE ABOVE:

If I suffer a condition from which there is no reasonable prospect of regaining the ability to think and act for myself, I want only care directed to my comfort and dignity, and authorize my agent to decline all treatment (including artificial nutrition and hydration) the primary purpose of which is to prolong my life.

If I suffer a condition from which there is no reasonable prospect of regaining the ability to think and act for myself, I want care directed to my comfort and dignity and also want artificial nutrition and hydration if needed, but authorize my agent to decline all other treatment the primary purpose of which is to prolong my life.

I want my life sustained by any reasonable medical measures, regardless of my condition.

In the event the person I appoint is unable, unwilling or unavailable to act as my health care agent, I hereby appoint _____ of _____ as alternate agent.

I hereby acknowledge that I have been provided with a disclosure statement explaining the effect of this document. I have read and understand the information contained in the disclosure statement.

The original of this document will be kept at _____ and the following persons and institutions shall have signed copies:

_____

_____

_____

In witness whereof, I have hereunto signed my name this _____ day of _____, 19 _____.

Signature _____

I declare that the principal appears to be of sound mind and free from duress at the time the durable power of attorney for health care is signed and that the principal has affirmed that he or she is aware of the nature of the document and is signing it freely and voluntarily.

Witness: _____

Address: _____

Telephone: _____

Witness: _____

Address: _____

Telephone: _____

Statement of ombudsman, hospital representative or other authorized person (to be signed only if the principal is in or is being admitted to a hospital, nursing home or residential care home):

I declare that I have personally explained the nature and effect of this durable power of attorney to the principal and that the principal understands the same.

Date: _____

Address: _____

Name: _____

Terminal Care Document (Living Will)

To my family, my physician, my lawyer, my clergyman. To any medical facility in whose care I happen to be. To any individual who may become responsible for my health, welfare or affairs.

Death is as much a reality as birth, growth, maturity and old age—it is the one certainty of life. If the time comes when I, _____, can no longer take part in decisions of my own future, let this statement stand as an expression of my wishes, while I am still of sound mind.

If the situation should arise in which I am in a terminal state and there is no reasonable expectation of my recovery, I direct that I be allowed to die a natural death and that my life not be prolonged by extraordinary measures. I do, however, ask that medication be mercifully administered to me to alleviate suffering even though this may shorten my remaining life.

This statement is made after careful consideration and is in accordance with my strong convictions and beliefs. I want the wishes and directions here expressed carried out to the extent permitted by law. Insofar as they are not legally enforceable, I hope that those to whom this will is addressed will regard themselves as morally bound by these provisions.

Signed: _____

Date: _____

Witness name _____ Witness name _____

Address _____ Address _____

Telephone _____ Telephone _____

Copies of this request have been given to:

_____

_____

_____

Advance Medical Directive

I, _____, willfully and voluntarily make known my desire and do hereby declare:

If at any time my attending physician should determine that I have a terminal condition where the application of life-prolonging procedures would serve only to artificially prolong the dying process, I direct that such procedures be withheld or withdrawn, and that I be permitted to die naturally with only the administration of medication or the performance of any medical procedure deemed necessary to provide me with comfort care or to alleviate pain (OPTION: I specifically direct that the following procedures or treatment be provided to me: _____)

In the absence of my ability to give directions regarding the use of such life-prolonging procedures, it is my intention that this declaration shall be honored by my family and physician as the final expression of my legal right to refuse medical or surgical treatment and accept the consequences of such refusal.

OPTION: APPOINTMENT OF AGENT (CROSS THROUGH IF YOU DO NOT WANT TO APPOINT AN AGENT TO MAKE HEALTH CARE DECISIONS FOR YOU.)

I hereby appoint _____ (primary agent), of _____ (address and telephone number), as my agent to make health care decisions on my behalf as authorized in this document. If _____ (primary agent) is not reasonably available or is unable or unwilling to act as my agent, then I appoint _____ (successor agent), of _____ (address and telephone number), to serve in that capacity.

I hereby grant to my agent, named above, full power and authority to make health care decisions on my behalf as described below whenever I have been determined to be incapable of making an informed decision about providing, withholding or withdrawing medical treatment. The phrase "incapable of making an informed decision" means unable to understand the nature, extent and probable consequences of a proposed medical decision or unable to make a rational evaluation of the risks and benefits of a proposed medical decision as compared with the risks and benefits of alternatives to that decision, or unable to communicate such understanding in any way. My agent's authority hereunder is effective as long as I am incapable of making an informed decision.

The determination that I am incapable of making an informed decision shall be made by my attending physician and a second physician or licensed clinical psychologist after a personal examination of me and shall be certified in writing. Such certification shall be required before treatment is withheld or withdrawn, and before, or as soon as reasonably practicable after, treatment is provided, and every 180 days thereafter while the treatment continues.

In exercising the power to make health care decisions on my behalf, my agent shall follow my desires and preferences as stated in this document or as otherwise known to my agent. My agent shall be guided by my medical diagnosis and prognosis and any information provided by my physicians as to the intrusiveness, pain, risks, and side effects associated with treatment or nontreatment. My agent shall not authorize a course of treatment which he knows, or upon reasonable inquiry ought to know, is contrary to my religious beliefs or my basic values, whether expressed orally or in writing. If my agent cannot determine what treatment choice I would have made on my own behalf, then my agent shall make a choice for me based on what he believes to be in my best interests.

Virginia

OPTION: POWERS OF MY AGENT (CROSS THROUGH ANY LANGUAGE YOU DO NOT WANT AND ADD ANY LANGUAGE YOU DO WANT)

The powers of my agent shall include the following:

A. To consent to or refuse or withdraw consent to any type of medical care, treatment, surgical procedure, diagnostic procedure, medication and the use of mechanical or other procedures that affect any bodily function, including, but not limited to, artificial respiration, artificially administered nutrition and hydration, and cardiopulmonary resuscitation. This authorization specifically includes the power to consent to the administration of dosages of pain relieving medication in excess of standard dosages in an amount sufficient to relieve pain, even if such medication carries the risk of addiction or inadvertently hastens my death;

B. To request, receive, and review any information, verbal or written, regarding my physical or mental health, including but not limited to, medical and hospital records, and to consent to the disclosure of this information;

C. To employ and discharge my health care providers;

D. To authorize my admission to or discharge (including transfer to another facility) from any hospital, hospice, nursing home, adult home or other medical care facility; and

E. To take any lawful actions that may be necessary to carry out these decisions, including the granting of releases of liability to medical providers.

F. Other statements: _____

_____

Further, my agent shall not be liable for the costs of treatment pursuant to his authorization, based solely on that authorization.

This advance directive shall not terminate in the event of my disability.

By signing below, I indicate that I am emotionally and mentally competent to make this advance directive and that I understand the purpose and effect of this document.

(Date) _____

(Signature of Declarant) _____

The declarant signed the foregoing advance directive in my presence. I am not the spouse or a blood relative of the declarant.

(Witness) _____

(Address) _____

(Telephone) _____

(Witness) _____

(Address) _____

(Telephone) _____

Health Care Directive

Directive made this _____ day of _____ (month, year).

I, _____, having the capacity to make health care decisions, willfully and voluntarily make known my desire that my dying shall not be artificially prolonged under the circumstances set forth below, and do hereby declare that:

(a) If at any time I should be diagnosed in writing to be in a terminal condition by the attending physician, or in a permanent unconscious condition by two physicians, and where the application of life-sustaining treatment would serve only to artificially prolong the process of my dying, I direct that such treatment be withheld or withdrawn, and that I be permitted to die naturally. I understand by using this form that a terminal condition means an incurable and irreversible condition caused by injury, disease, or illness, that would within reasonable medical judgment cause death within a reasonable period of time in accordance with accepted medical standards, and where the application of life-sustaining treatment would serve only to prolong the process of dying. I further understand in using this form that a permanent unconscious condition means an incurable and irreversible condition in which I am medically assessed within reasonable medical judgment as having no reasonable probability of recovery from an irreversible coma or a persistent vegetative state.

(b) In the absence of my ability to give directions regarding the use of such life-sustaining treatment, it is my intention that this directive shall be honored by my family and physician(s) as the final expression of my legal right to refuse medical or surgical treatment and I accept the consequences of such refusal. If another person is appointed to make these decisions for me, whether through a durable power of attorney or otherwise, I request that the person be guided by this directive and any other clear expressions of my desires.

(c) If I am diagnosed to be in a terminal condition or in a permanent unconscious condition (check one);
I DO want to have artificially provided nutrition and hydration.
I DO NOT want to have artificially provided nutrition and hydration.

(d) If I have been diagnosed as pregnant and that diagnosis is known to my physician, this directive shall have no force or effect during the course of my pregnancy.

(e) I understand the full import of this directive and I am emotionally and mentally capable to make the health care decisions contained in this directive.

(f) I understand that before I sign this directive, I can add to or delete from or otherwise change the wording of this directive and that I may add to or delete from this directive at any time and that any changes shall be consistent with Washington state law or federal constitutional law to be legally valid.

(g) It is my wish that every part of this directive be fully implemented. If for any reason any part is held invalid it is my wish that the remainder of my directive be implemented.

Signed _____

City, County and State of Residence _____

The declarer has been personally known to me and I believe him or her to be capable of making health care decisions.

Witness name: _____   Witness name: _____

Address: _____   Address: _____

Telephone: _____   Telephone: _____

Medical Power of Attorney

Dated: _____, 19_____.

    I, _____, (insert your name and address), hereby appoint _____ (insert the name, address, area code and telephone number of the person you wish to designate as your representative) as my representative to act on my behalf to give, withhold or withdraw informed consent to health care decisions in the event that I am not able to do so myself. If my representative is unable, unwilling or disqualified to serve, then I appoint _____ as my successor representative.

    This appointment shall extend to (but not be limited to) decisions relating to medical treatment, surgical treatment, nursing care, medication, hospitalization, care and treatment in a nursing home or other facility, and home health care. The representative appointed by this document is specifically authorized to act on my behalf to consent to, refuse or withdraw any and all medical treatment or diagnostic procedures, if my representative determines that I, if able to do so, would consent to, refuse or withdraw such treatment or procedures. Such authority shall include, but not be limited to, the withholding or withdrawal of life-prolonging intervention when in the opinion of two physicians who have examined me, one of whom is my attending physician, such life-prolonging intervention offers no medical hope of benefit.

    I appoint this representative because I believe this person understands my wishes and values and will act to carry into effect the health care decisions that I would make if I were able to do so, and because I also believe that this person will act in my best interests when my wishes are unknown. It is my intent that my family, my physician and all legal authorities be bound by the decisions that are made by the representative appointed by this document, and it is my intent that these decisions should not be the subject of review by any health care provider, or administrative or judicial agency.

    It is my intent that this document be legally binding and effective. In the event that the law does not recognize this document as legally binding and effective, it is my intent that this document be taken as a formal statement of my desire concerning the method by which any health care decisions should be made on my behalf during the period when I am unable to make such decisions.

    In exercising the authority under this medical power of attorney, my representative shall act consistently with my special directives or limitations as stated below:

SPECIAL DIRECTIVES OR LIMITATIONS ON THIS POWER: (If none, write "none.")

_____

_____

_____

    THIS MEDICAL POWER OF ATTORNEY SHALL BECOME EFFECTIVE ONLY UPON MY INCAPACITY TO GIVE, WITHHOLD OR WITHDRAW INFORMED CONSENT TO MY OWN MEDICAL CARE.

    These directives shall supersede any directives made in any previously executed document concerning my health care.

X _____
Signature of Principal

West Virginia

I did not sign the principal's signature above. I am at least eighteen years of age and am not related to the principal by blood or marriage. I am not entitled to any portion of the estate of the principal according to the laws of intestate succession of the state of the principal's domicile or to the best of my knowledge under any will of the principal or codicil thereto, or legally responsible for the costs of the principal's medical or other care. I am not the principal's attending physician, nor am I the representative or successor representative of the principal.

WITNESS: _____

ADDRESS: _____

TELEPHONE: _____

DATE: _____

WITNESS: _____

ADDRESS: _____

TELEPHONE: _____

DATE: _____

STATE OF _____,
COUNTY OF _____,
to-wit:

I, _____, a Notary Public of said County, do certify that _____, as principal, and _____ and _____, as witnesses, whose names are signed to the writing above bearing date on the _____ day of _____, 19_____, have this day acknowledged the same before me.

Given under my hand this _____ day of _____, 19 ____.

My commission expires: _____

Notary Public _____

Living Will

Living will made this _____ day of _____ (month, year). I, _____, being of sound mind, willfully and voluntarily declare that in the absence of my ability to give directions regarding the use of life-prolonging intervention, it is my desire that my dying shall not be artificially prolonged under the following circumstances:

"If at any time I should be certified by two physicians who have personally examined me, one of whom is my attending physician, to have a terminal condition or to be in a persistent vegetative state, I direct that life-prolonging intervention that would serve solely to artificially prolong the dying process or maintain me in a persistent vegetative state be withheld or withdrawn, and that I be permitted to die naturally with only the administration of medication or the performance of any other procedure deemed necessary to keep me comfortable and alleviate pain.

SPECIAL DIRECTIVE OR LIMITATIONS ON THIS DECLARATION: (If none, write "none".)

"It is my intention that this living will be honored as the final expression of my legal right to refuse medical or surgical treatment and accept the consequences resulting from such refusal.

I understand the full import of this living will.

Signed _____

Address _____

_____

"I did not sign the declarant's signature above for or at the direction of the declarant. I am at least eighteen years of age and am not related to the declarant by blood or marriage, entitled to any portion of the estate of the declarant according to the laws of intestate succession of the state of the declarant's domicile or to the best of my knowledge under any will of declarant or codicil thereto, or directly financially responsible for declarant's medical care. I am not the declarant's attending physician or the declarant's health care representative, proxy or successor health care representative under a medical power of attorney.

Witness _____   Witness _____

Address _____   Address _____

Telephone _____   Telephone _____

STATE OF _____

COUNTY OF _____

The foregoing instrument was acknowledged before me this _____ (date) by the declarant and by the two witnesses whose signatures appear above.

My commission expires: _____

Signature of Notary Public: _____

"Notice to Person Making This Document

YOU HAVE THE RIGHT TO MAKE DECISIONS ABOUT YOUR HEALTH CARE. NO HEALTH CARE MAY BE GIVEN TO YOU OVER YOUR OBJECTION, AND NECESSARY HEALTH CARE MAY NOT BE STOPPED OR WITHHELD IF YOU OBJECT.

BECAUSE YOUR HEALTH CARE PROVIDERS IN SOME CASES MAY NOT HAVE HAD THE OPPORTUNITY TO ESTABLISH A LONG-TERM RELATIONSHIP WITH YOU, THEY ARE OFTEN UNFAMILIAR WITH YOUR BELIEFS AND VALUES AND THE DETAILS OF YOUR FAMILY RELATIONSHIPS. THIS POSES A PROBLEM IF YOU BECOME PHYSICALLY OR MENTALLY UNABLE TO MAKE DECISIONS ABOUT YOUR HEALTH CARE.

IN ORDER TO AVOID THIS PROBLEM, YOU MAY SIGN THIS LEGAL DOCUMENT TO SPECIFY THE PERSON WHOM YOU WANT TO MAKE HEALTH CARE DECISIONS FOR YOU IF YOU ARE UNABLE TO MAKE THOSE DECISIONS PERSONALLY. THAT PERSON IS KNOWN AS YOUR HEALTH CARE AGENT. YOU SHOULD TAKE SOME TIME TO DISCUSS YOUR THOUGHTS AND BELIEFS ABOUT MEDICAL TREATMENT WITH THE PERSON OR PERSONS WHOM YOU HAVE SPECIFIED. YOU MAY STATE IN THIS DOCUMENT ANY TYPES OF HEALTH CARE THAT YOU DO OR DO NOT DESIRE, AND YOU MAY LIMIT THE AUTHORITY OF YOUR HEALTH CARE AGENT. IF YOUR HEALTH CARE AGENT IS UNAWARE OF YOUR DESIRES WITH RESPECT TO A PARTICULAR HEALTH CARE DECISION, HE OR SHE IS REQUIRED TO DETERMINE WHAT WOULD BE IN YOUR BEST INTERESTS IN MAKING THE DECISION.

THIS IS AN IMPORTANT LEGAL DOCUMENT. IT GIVES YOUR AGENT BROAD POWERS TO MAKE HEALTH CARE DECISIONS FOR YOU. IT REVOKES ANY PRIOR POWER OF ATTORNEY FOR HEALTH CARE THAT YOU MAY HAVE MADE. IF YOU WISH TO CHANGE YOUR POWER OF ATTORNEY FOR HEALTH CARE, YOU MAY REVOKE THIS DOCUMENT AT ANY TIME BY DESTROYING IT, BY DIRECTING ANOTHER PERSON TO DESTROY IT IN YOUR PRESENCE, BY SIGNING A WRITTEN AND DATED STATEMENT OR BY STATING THAT IT IS REVOKED IN THE PRESENCE OF TWO WITNESSES. IF YOU REVOKE, YOU SHOULD NOTIFY YOUR AGENT, YOUR HEALTH CARE PROVIDERS AND ANY OTHER PERSON TO WHOM YOU HAVE GIVEN A COPY. IF YOUR AGENT IS YOUR SPOUSE AND YOUR MARRIAGE IS ANNULLED OR YOU ARE DIVORCED AFTER SIGNING THIS DOCUMENT, THE DOCUMENT IS INVALID.

DO NOT SIGN THIS DOCUMENT UNLESS YOU CLEARLY UNDERSTAND IT.

IT IS SUGGESTED THAT YOU KEEP THE ORIGINAL OF THIS DOCUMENT ON FILE WITH YOUR PHYSICIAN."

Wisconsin

POWER OF ATTORNEY FOR HEALTH CARE

Document made this _____ day of _____ (month) _____ (year).

CREATION OF POWER OF ATTORNEY FOR HEALTH CARE

I, _____ (print name, address and date of birth), being of sound mind, intend by this document to create a power of attorney for health care. My executing this power of attorney for health care is voluntary. Despite the creation of this power of attorney for health care, I expect to be fully informed about and allowed to participate in any health care decision for me, to the extent that I am able. For the purposes of this document, "health care decision" means an informed decision to accept, maintain, discontinue or refuse any care, treatment, service or procedure to maintain, diagnose or treat my physical or mental condition.

DESIGNATION OF HEALTH CARE AGENT

If I am no longer able to make health care decisions for myself, due to my incapacity, I hereby designate _____ (print name, address and telephone number) to be my health care agent for the purpose of making health care decisions on my behalf. If he or she is ever unable or unwilling to do so, I hereby designate _____ (print name, address and telephone number) to be my alternate health care agent for the purpose of making health care decisions on my behalf. Neither my health care agent or my alternate health care agent whom I have designated is my health care provider, an employee of my health care provider, an employee of a health care facility in which I am a patient or a spouse of any of those persons, unless he or she is also my relative. For purposes of this document, "incapacity" exists if 2 physicians or a physician and a psychologist who have personally examined me sign a statement that specifically expresses their opinion that I have a condition that means that I am unable to receive and evaluate information effectively or to communicate decisions to such an extent that I lack the capacity to manage my health care decisions. A copy of that statement must be attached to this document.

GENERAL STATEMENT OF AUTHORITY GRANTED

Unless I have specified otherwise in this document, if I ever have incapacity I instruct my health care provider to obtain the health care decision of my health care agent, if I need treatment, for all of my health care and treatment. I have discussed my desires thoroughly with my health care agent and believe that he or she understands my philosophy regarding the health care decisions I would make if I were so able. I desire that my wishes be carried out through the authority given to my health care agent under this document.

If I am unable, due to my incapacity, to make a health care decision, my health care agent is instructed to make the health care decision for me, but my health care agent should try to discuss with me any specific proposed health care if I am able to communicate in any manner, including by blinking my eyes. If this communication cannot be made, my health care agent shall base his or her decision on any health care choices that I have expressed prior to the time of the decision. If I have not expressed a health care choice about the health care in question and communication cannot be made, my health care agent shall base his or her health care decision on what he or she believes to be in my best interest.

LIMITATIONS ON MENTAL HEALTH TREATMENT

My health care agent may not admit or commit me on an inpatient basis to an institution for mental disease, an intermediate care facility for the mentally retarded, a state treatment facility or a treatment facility. My health care agent may not consent to experimental mental health research or psychosurgery, electroconvulsive treatment or drastic mental health treatment procedures for me.

ADMISSION TO NURSING HOMES OR COMMUNITY-BASED RESIDENTIAL FACILITIES

My health care agent may admit me to a nursing home or community-based residential facility for short-term stays for recuperative care or respite care.

If I have checked "Yes" to the following, my health care agent may admit me for a purpose other than recuperative care or respite care, but if I have checked "No" to the following, my health care agent may not so admit me:

1. A nursing home—Yes _____ No _____

2. A community-based residential facility—Yes _____ No _____

If I have not checked either "Yes" or "No" immediately above, my health care agent may only admit me for short-term stays for recuperative care or respite care.

PROVISION OF A FEEDING TUBE

If I have checked "Yes" to the following, my health care agent may have a feeding tube withheld or withdrawn from me, unless my physician has advised that, in his or her professional judgment, this will cause me pain or will reduce my comfort. If I have checked "No" to the following, my health care agent may not have a feeding tube withheld or withdrawn from me.

My health care agent may not have orally ingested nutrition or hydration withheld or withdrawn from me unless provision of the nutrition or hydration is medically contraindicated.

Withhold or withdraw a feeding tube —Yes _____ No _____

If I have not checked either "Yes" or "No" immediately above, my health care agent may not have a feeding tube withdrawn from me.

HEALTH CARE DECISIONS FOR PREGNANT WOMEN

If I have checked "Yes" to the following, my health care agent may make health care decisions for me even if my agent knows I am pregnant. If I have checked "No" to the following, my health care agent may not make health care decisions for me if my health care agent knows I am pregnant.

Health care decisions if I am pregnant—Yes _____ No _____

If I have not checked either "Yes" or "No" immediately above, my health care agent may not make health care decisions for me if my health care agent knows I am pregnant.

STATEMENT OF DESIRES, SPECIAL PROVISIONS OR LIMITATIONS

In exercising authority under this document, my health care agent shall act consistently with my following stated desires, if any, and is subject to any special provisions or limitations that I specify. The following are any specific desires, provisions or limitations that I wish to state (add more items if needed):

1) _____

2) _____

3) _____

INSPECTION AND DISCLOSURE OF INFORMATION RELATING TO MY PHYSICAL OR MENTAL HEALTH

Subject to any limitations in this document, my health care agent has the authority to do all of the following:

(a) Request, review and receive any information, verbal or written, regarding my physical or mental health, including medical and hospital records.

Wisconsin

(b) Execute on my behalf any documents that may be required in order to obtain this information.

(c) Consent to the disclosure of this information.

(The principal and the witnesses all must sign the document at the same time.)

SIGNATURE OF PRINCIPAL

(person creating the power of attorney for health care)

Signature _____

Date _____

(The signing of this document by the principal revokes all previous powers of attorney for health care documents.)

Signature _____

Date _____

STATEMENT OF WITNESSES

I know the principal personally and I believe him or her to be of sound mind and at least 18 years of age. I believe that his or her execution of this power of attorney for health care is voluntary. I am at least 18 years of age and am not related to the principal by blood, marriage or adoption, and am not directly financially responsible for the principal's health care. I am not a health care provider who is serving the principal at this time, an employee of the health care provider; other than a chaplain or a social worker, or an employee, other than a chaplain or a social worker, of an inpatient inpatient health care facility in which the declarant is a patient. I am not the principal's health care agent. To the best of my knowledge, I am not entitled to and do not have a claim on the principal's estate.

Witness No. 1: _____

(print) Name _____

Address _____

Date _____

Witness No. 2: _____

(print) Name _____

Address _____

Date _____

STATEMENT OF HEALTH CARE AGENT AND
ALTERNATE HEALTH CARE AGENT

I understand that _____ (name of principal) has designated me to be his or her health care agent or alternate health care agent if he or she is ever found to have incapacity and unable to make health care decisions himself or herself. _____ (name of principal) has discussed his or her desires regarding health care decisions with me.

Agent's signature _____

Address _____

Alternate's signature _____

Address _____

Failure to execute a power of attorney for health care document under chapter 155 of the Wisconsin Statutes creates no presumption about the intent of any individual with regard to his or her health care decisions.

This power of attorney for health care is executed as provided in chapter 155 of the Wisconsin Statutes.

Declaration to Physicians

1. I, _____, being of sound mind, voluntarily state my desire that my dying may not be prolonged under the circumstances specified in this document. Under those circumstances, I direct that I be permitted to die naturally.

If I am unable to give directions regarding the use of life-sustaining procedures or feeding tubes, I intend that my family and physician honor this document as the final expression of my legal right to refuse medical or surgical treatment and to accept the consequences from this refusal.

2. If I have a TERMINAL CONDITION, as determined by 2 physicians who have personally examined me, I do not want my dying to be artifically prolonged and I do not want life-sustaining procedures to be used. In addition, if I have such a terminal condition, the following are my directions regarding the use of feeding tubes (check only one).

    a. Use feeding tubes if I have a terminal condition _____

    b. Do not use feeding tubes if I have a terminal condition _____

    c. If I have not checked either box, feeding tubes will be used.

3. If I am in a PERSISTENT VEGETATIVE STATE, as determined by 2 physicians who have personally examined me, the following are my directions regarding the use of life-sustaining procedures and feeding tubes:

    a. Check only one:

    Use life-sustaining procedures if I am in a persistent vegetative state _____

    Do no use life-sustaining procedures if I am in a persistent vegetative state _____

    If I have not checked either box, life-sustaining procedures will be used.

    b. Check only one:

    Use feeding tubes if I am in a persistent vegetative state _____

    Do not use feeding tubes if I am in a persistent vegetative state _____

    If I have not checked either box, feeding tubes will be used.

4. By law, this document cannot be used to authorize: a) withholding or withdrawal of any medication, procedure or feeding tube if to do so would cause me pain or reduce my comfort; and b) withholding or withdrawal of nutrition or hydration that is administered to me through means other than a feeding tube unless, in my physician's opinion, this administration is medically contraindicated.

5. If I have been diagnosed as pregnant and my physician knows of this diagnosis, this document has no effect during the course of my pregnancy.

Signed _____

Date _____

Address _____

I know the person signing this document personally and I believe him or her to be of sound mind. I am not related to the person signing this document by blood, marriage or adoption, and am not entitled to and do not have a claim on any portion of the person's estate and am not otherwise restricted by law from being a witness.

Witness _____

Witness _____

WYOMING

Declaration

Declaration made this _____ day of _____ (month, year). I, _____, being of sound mind, willfully and voluntarily make known my desire that my dying shall not be artificially prolonged under the circumstances set forth below, do hereby declare:

If at any time I should have an incurable injury, disease or other illness certified to be a terminal condition by two (2) physicians who have personally examined me, one (1) of whom shall be my attending physician, and the physicians have determined that my death will occur whether or not life-sustaining procedures are utilized and where the application of life-sustaining procedures would serve only to artificially prolong the dying process, I direct that such procedures be withheld or withdrawn, and that I be permitted to die naturally with only the administration of medication or the performance of any medical procedure deemed necessary to provide me with comfort care. If, in spite of this declaration, I am comatose or otherwise unable to make treatment decisions for myself, I HEREBY designate _____ to make treatment decisions for me.

In the absence of my ability to give directions regarding the use of life-sustaining procedures, it is my intention that this declaration shall be honored by my family and physician(s) and agent as the final expression of my legal right to refuse medical or surgical treatment and accept the consequences from this refusal. I understand the full import of this declaration and I am emotionally and mentally competent to make this declaration.

Signed _____

City, County and State of Residence _____

The declarant has been personally known to me and I believe him or her to be of sound mind. I did not sign the declarant's signature above for or at the direction of the declarant. I am not related to the declarant by blood or marriage, entitled to any portion of the estate of the declarant according to the laws of intestate succession or under any will of the declarant or codicil thereto, or directly financially responsible for declarant's medical care.

Witness _____   Witness _____

Address _____   Address _____

Telephone _____   Telephone _____

NOTICE

This document has significant medical, legal and possible ethical implications and effects. Before you sign this document, you should become completely familiar with these implications and effects. The operation, effects and implications of this document may be discussed with a physician, a lawyer or a clergyman of your choice.